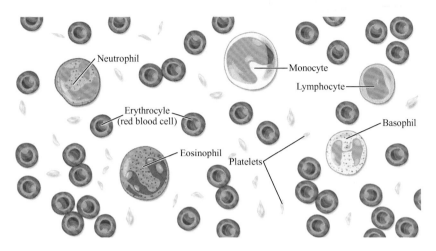

Fig 5.1   The cells and cellular components of human blood

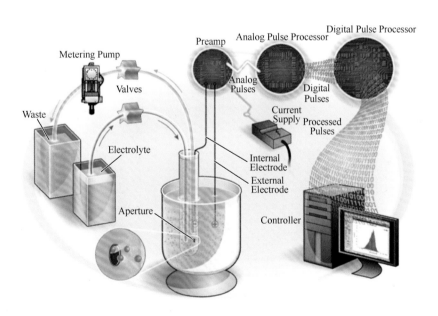

Fig 5.2   The passage of a cell through an aperture

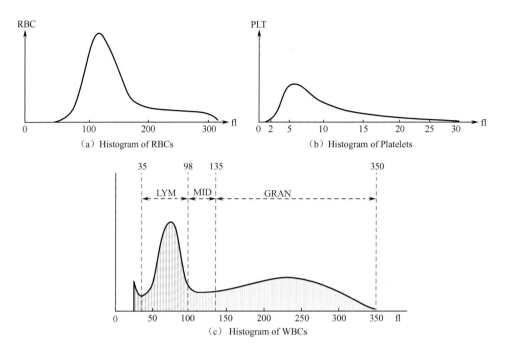

(a) Histogram of RBCs

(b) Histogram of Platelets

(c) Histogram of WBCs

Fig 5.5　Histograms of the cells

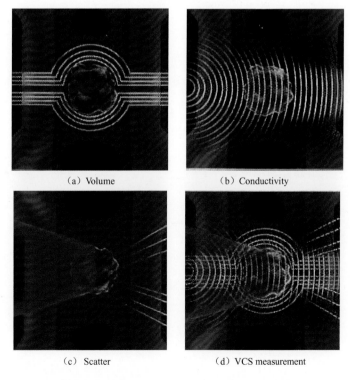

(a) Volume

(b) Conductivity

(c) Scatter

(d) VCS measurement

Fig 5.6　Volume, conductivity and scatter technology

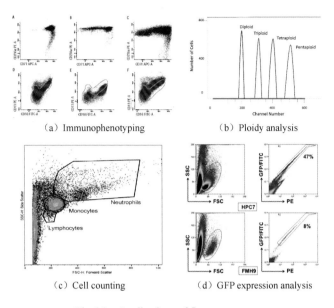

（a）Immunophenotyping　　　　　（b）Ploidy analysis

（c）Cell counting　　　　　（d）GFP expression analysis

Fig 6.1　Applications of flow cytometers

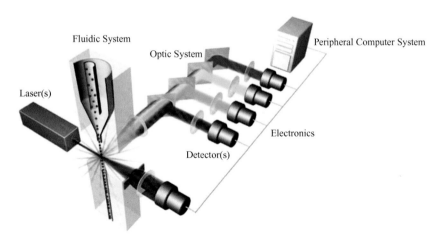

Fig 6.2　Primary systems of the flow cytometer

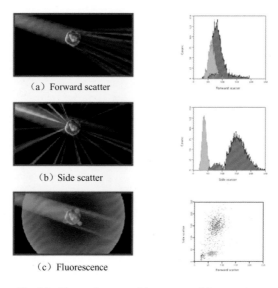

（a）Forward scatter

（b）Side scatter

（c）Fluorescence

Fig 6.4   Forward scatter, side scatter and fluorescence

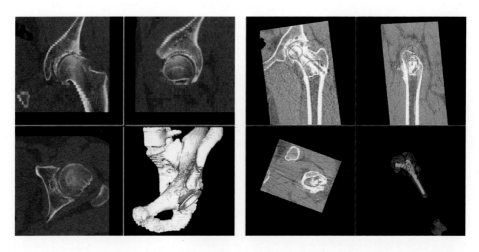

Fig 9.3   Applications of image-guided surgery: planning of the cup implant; planning of the femoral implant

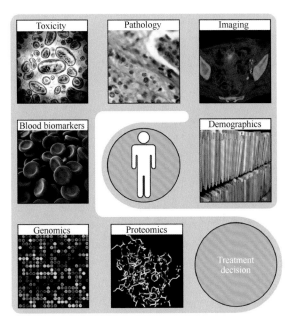

Fig 11.1　Different sources of information, e.g. demographics, imaging, pathology, toxicity, biomarkers, genomics and proteomics, can be used for selecting the optimal treatment

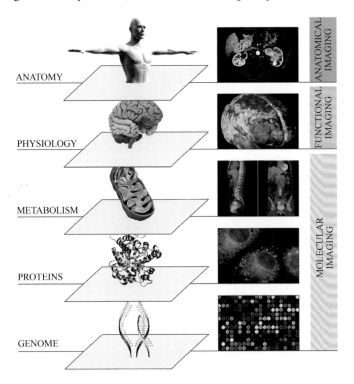

Fig 11.2　Multilevel imaging: anatomical, functional, and molecular imaging

(a)　　　　　　　　(b)　　　　　　　　(c)

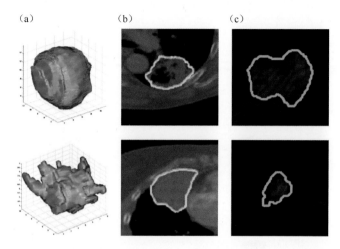

Fig 11.3　(a) Two representative 3D representations of a round tumour (top) and spiky tumour (bottom) measured by computed tomography (CT) imaging. (b) Texture differences between non-small cell lung cancer (NSCLC) tumours measured using CT imaging, more heterogeneous (top) and more homogeneous (bottom). (c) Differences of FDG-PET uptake, showing heterogeneous uptake

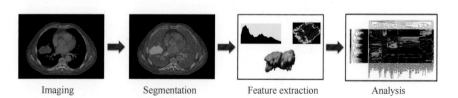

Imaging　　　　　　Segmentation　　　　Feature extraction　　　　Analysis

Fig 11.4　The radiomics workflow

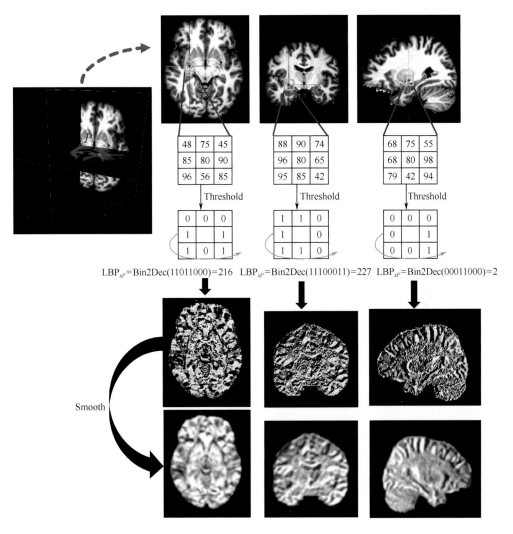

$\text{LBP}_{xP} = \text{Bin2Dec}(11011000) = 216 \quad \text{LBP}_{xP} = \text{Bin2Dec}(11100011) = 227 \quad \text{LBP}_{xP} = \text{Bin2Dec}(00011000) = 2$

Smooth

Fig 11.6   A brief illustration of the calculation of LBP-TOP value in pixel P in the axial, coronal, and sagittal orientations. Pixel P is denoted by the red color, with its 363 neighborhoods circled by a yellow square in the 2D plane. Bin2Dec is a function for transferring binary code to decimal values

教育部高等学校生物医学工程类专业教学指导委员会"十四五"规划教材

专业英语
（生物医学工程领域）

严荣国　闫士举　王殊轶　陈丽雯　贺　晨　编著

电子工业出版社

Publishing House of Electronics Industry

北京·BEIJING

内 容 简 介

本教材适用于生物医学工程领域的专业英语教学。生物医学工程是一门理、工、医相结合的新兴交叉学科，涉及的知识和范围非常广泛。绪论部分介绍生物医学工程领域专业英语的词汇特点、句法特点和翻译技巧。第一部分介绍生物医学工程的通用描述（General Descriptions on Biomedical Engineering），包括生物医学工程基本概念、生物工程与生物医学工程的区别、生物医学传感器和生物医学仪器、医疗器械，以及细胞层次上的血细胞分析技术等；第二部分介绍从本学科诸位老师的科研方向汲取的若干个典型案例（Special Topics on Biomedical Engineering），这一部分从机械、电子、图像处理、人因工程等不同侧面，介绍了生物医学工程的典型应用；针对研究生发表学术论文的需求，第三部分介绍如何准备英文论文（About Submitting a Paper）。

本教材内容涵盖生物医学工程领域中的众多方面，贴近时代前沿、知识面广、难度适中。本书可作为普通高等学校生物医学工程领域的本科生及研究生的专业英语教材，也可作为相关工程技术人员学习和提升专业英语的参考用书。

图书在版编目（CIP）数据

专业英语：生物医学工程领域 / 严荣国等编著. —北京：电子工业出版社，2023.7

ISBN 978-7-121-45753-1

Ⅰ. ①专… Ⅱ. ①严… Ⅲ. ①生物医学工程－英语－教材 Ⅳ. ①R318

中国国家版本馆 CIP 数据核字（2023）第 103802 号

责任编辑：张小乐

印　　刷：涿州市京南印刷厂

装　　订：涿州市京南印刷厂

出版发行：电子工业出版社

　　　　　北京市海淀区万寿路 173 信箱　　邮编 100036

开　　本：720×1 000　1/16　印张：11.75　字数：356 千字　彩插：4

版　　次：2023 年 7 月第 1 版

印　　次：2023 年 7 月第 1 次印刷

定　　价：45.00 元

凡所购买电子工业出版社图书有缺损问题，请向购买书店调换。若书店售缺，请与本社发行部联系，联系及邮购电话：（010）88254888，88258888。

质量投诉请发邮件至 zlts@phei.com.cn，盗版侵权举报请发邮件至 dbqq@phei.com.cn。

本书咨询联系方式：（010）88254462，zhxl@phei.com.cn。

前　言

生物医学工程是一门综合生命科学和工程技术，理、工、医相结合的新兴交叉学科，体现了新知识的综合和发展，对提高医学水平、促进医学科学的现代化发挥着关键性的作用。生物医学工程学科的典型特点是多学科交叉与融合，其主要涵盖领域有生物信息学、生物材料、组织工程、医疗器械、医学成像、临床工程、康复工程、生物力学等。

我国生物医学工程学科的普及、教学和科研水平尚不及欧美发达国家，要在这一领域赶超世界先进水平，关键就在于我们的高等教育要面向世界，与国际先进水平接轨，培养既有扎实的基础理论知识，又有较强的解决实际问题能力及创新思维的人才。

全书共 13 个单元（Unit），每个单元均包含 Text、Words and Expressions、Key Sentences 和 Further Readings 四个部分。Text 部分是课堂教学的主体内容，Words and Expressions 给出了 Text 里面出现的重点单词和词组，Key Sentences 给出了重点句子的解析，而 Further Readings 提供了与该单元主题有关的课外阅读材料。

本教材建设项目获得了上海理工大学研究生院的资助，本书由复旦大学聚合物分子工程国家重点实验室纪岱宗主审，上海理工大学健康科学与工程学院刘宝林教授对本书的总体策划和编排提出了许多建设性的意见。各章分别由上海理工大学健康科学与工程学院严荣国（绪论，Unit 1、3、4、5、6、8、13）、闫士举（Unit 9、10、11）、贺晨（Unit 7）、陈丽雯（Unit 2）和王殊轶（Unit 12）整理。

本书部分英文资料来源于网络，均在参考文献中加以标注。本书可作为生物医学工程专业本科生和研究生的教材或教学参考书，也可用作相关领域人员提高英文写作水平、参与国际学术交流活动的参考书。

由于时间和编者水平有限，书中难免有不足、错漏和不妥之处，敬请读者批评指正。

编　著　者

目　　录

绪论　专业英语的特点 ……………………………………………………………… 1

专业英语的词汇特点 ……………………………………………………………… 1

专业英语的句法特点 ……………………………………………………………… 6

专业英语翻译技巧 ………………………………………………………………… 8

Part I　General Descriptions on Biomedical Engineering …………………………… 12

Unit 1　Introduction to Biomedical Engineering …………………………………… 12

1.1　Bioinformatics ……………………………………………………………… 13

1.2　Biomaterial ………………………………………………………………… 14

1.3　Tissue Engineering ………………………………………………………… 14

1.4　Medical Devices …………………………………………………………… 15

1.5　Medical Imaging …………………………………………………………… 15

1.6　Clinical Engineering ……………………………………………………… 15

1.7　Rehabilitation Engineering ………………………………………………… 16

1.8　Biomechanics ……………………………………………………………… 16

Words and Expressions ………………………………………………………… 16

Key Sentences …………………………………………………………………… 18

Further Readings ………………………………………………………………… 19

Unit 2　Differences Between Bioengineering and Biomedical Engineering …………… 25

2.1　Research Areas …………………………………………………………… 25

2.2　Education and Personal Needs …………………………………………… 26

2.3　Job Duties ………………………………………………………………… 27

2.4　Job Outlook ………………………………………………………………… 27

Words and Expressions ………………………………………………………… 28

Key Sentences …………………………………………………………………… 28

Further Readings ………………………………………………………………… 29

Unit 3　Biomedical Sensors and Biomedical Instrumentation ……………………… 32

3.1　Definition of a Sensor ……………………………………………………… 32

3.2　Classifying Sensors ………………………………………………………… 32

3.3　Biomedical Sensors ………………………………………………………… 32

3.4　Biomedical Instrumentation ……………………………………………… 34

Words and Expressions ………………………………………………………… 36

Key Sentences …………………………………………………………………… 37

Further Readings ………………………………………………………………… 37

Unit 4　Fundamentals of Medical Devices···40
　　4.1　Definition of Medical Devices in the United States·······················40
　　4.2　Definition of Medical Devices in China ·································41
　　4.3　Types of Medical Devices ··42
　　4.4　List of Some Medical Devices ·····································43
　　Words and Expressions ··46
　　Key Sentences ···48
　　Further Readings ···49

Unit 5　Introduction to Hematology Analysis ···53
　　5.1　Cellular Analysis Using the Coulter Principle ·························54
　　5.2　VCS Technology···56
　　Words and Expressions ··58
　　Key Sentences ···59
　　Further Readings ···60

Unit 6　Introduction to Flow Cytometry ··63
　　6.1　Definition of Flow Cytometry·······································63
　　6.2　Primary Systems of Flow Cytometer ·································64
　　6.3　Interrogation Point ··64
　　6.4　Hydrodynamic Focusing ··64
　　6.5　Size Comparison ···65
　　6.6　Forward Scatter··65
　　6.7　Detector for Forward Scatter ····································66
　　6.8　Forward Scatter Histogram ·····································66
　　6.9　Side Scatter Histogram ··66
　　6.10　Scatter Plot···66
　　6.11　2D Scatter Plot of Blood·······································67
　　6.12　Energy State Diagram···67
　　6.13　Fluorescent Light ··67
　　6.14　Fluorescence Detection ·······································67
　　6.15　Fluorescence One Color Histogram ·······························68
　　6.16　Two-Color Experiment, Spectra Compatible····························68
　　6.17　Two-Color Dot Plot ···68
　　6.18　Filters Collect Two Colors ·····································68
　　6.19　Emission Filter Types ···69
　　6.20　Threshold for Forward Scatter····································69
　　6.21　Summary··69

Words and Expressions ·· 70

Key Sentences ··· 71

Further Readings ·· 72

Unit 7　Introduction to Limb Prostheses·· 77

　　7.1　Upper Limb Prostheses··· 77

　　　　7.1.1　Prosthetic Hands and Tools ··· 78

　　　　7.1.2　Adjustable and Static Devices ··· 78

　　　　7.1.3　Body-Powered Upper Limb Prostheses·· 78

　　　　7.1.4　Externally Powered Upper Limb Prostheses ····································· 79

　　7.2　Lower Limb Prostheses ··· 80

　　　　7.2.1　Mechanically Passive Devices ·· 81

　　　　7.2.2　Active Lower Limb Devices·· 82

　　　　7.2.3　Prescription of a Prosthesis ·· 83

Words and Expressions ·· 83

Key Sentences ··· 84

Further Readings ·· 85

Part II　Special Topics on Biomedical Engineering ·· 87

Unit 8　Introduction to Bluetooth Enabled FootFit Device ·································· 87

　　8.1　Summary of Study Protocol ·· 88

　　8.2　Overview of the System··· 89

　　8.3　Nine Prescribed Exercises ··· 93

Words and Expressions ·· 94

Key Sentences ··· 94

Further Readings ·· 95

Unit 9　Computer-Assisted Orthopaedic Surgery ··· 98

　　9.1　Basics of Computer-Assisted Orthopaedic Surgery······································ 98

　　9.2　CT-Based Navigation Systems·· 102

Words and Expressions ··· 105

Key Sentences ·· 106

Further Readings ··· 107

Unit 10　Minimally Invasive Surgery and Navigation: Total Knee Arthroplasty ··········· 110

　　10.1　The Surgetics Bone-Morphing System··· 110

　　10.2　Principles of MIS in Total Knee Arthroplasty··· 113

Words and Expressions ··· 116

Key Sentences ·· 117

Further Readings ··· 117

Unit 11　Medical Image-Based Disease Prediction ··· 121

    11.1　Computer-Assisted Diagnosis and Radiomics ·· 121

    11.2　Medical Image-Based Alzheimer Disease Prediction ··································· 124

    Words and Expressions ··· 128

    Key Sentences ·· 129

    Further Readings ··· 130

Unit 12　Human Factors Engineering: Design of Medical Devices ··························· 134

    12.1　Introduction of Human Factors Engineering ·· 134

    12.2　HFE Medical Device Design ··· 135

        12.2.1　Seek User Input ·· 135

        12.2.2　Establish Design Priorities··· 136

        12.2.3　Accommodate User Characteristics and Capabilities ······················· 139

        12.2.4　Accommodate Users' Needs and Preferences ······························· 142

    Words and Expressions ··· 144

    Key Sentences ·· 145

    Further Readings ··· 145

Part III　About Submitting a Paper ··· 149

Unit 13　Considering About Preparing a Paper ·· 149

    13.1　Types of Papers ··· 149

    13.2　Choice to Publish Open Access ··· 150

    13.3　Use of Inclusive Language ·· 150

    13.4　Article Structure ·· 150

    13.5　Role of the Funding Source ··· 151

    13.6　Declaration of Interest ··· 152

    13.7　Peer Review ··· 152

    13.8　General Steps to Prepare a Journal Paper ·· 152

    13.9　Online Submission ··· 154

    13.10　Publication Policy·· 154

    13.11　Plagiarism Policy ·· 154

    Words and Expressions ··· 155

    Key Sentences ·· 155

    Further Readings ··· 156

附录 A　主要学术机构 ··· 158

附录 B　常用英文期刊列表 ··· 162

附录 C　常用中文期刊列表 ··· 165

附录 D　词汇表 ··· 166

参考文献 ·· 179

绪论　专业英语的特点

专业英语是科技人员在世界范围内进行科学技术交流的重要工具，是自然科学和技术人员从事专业活动时所使用的一种文体，常见于科学著作、学术论文、实验报告、产品说明书等。

与新闻报刊、日常交流用语不同，专业英语特色鲜明，不追求语言的艺术美，而是讲究逻辑清晰、条理清楚、叙述准确，具有行文简洁、陈述客观、结构严密、强调事实、专业性强等特点。

一方面，专业英语的翻译是一门科学而不是艺术，不需要大量的再创作，需要的是译者能够准确、客观地翻译原文所表达的专业知识。总体来说，专业英语的文体特点可以通过构词、句法、修辞等层面表现出来。

另一方面，生物医学工程是结合物理、化学、数学和计算机与工程学原理，从事生物学、医学、行为学或卫生学等研究的学科，研究成果用于疾病预防、诊断和治疗，患者康复，卫生状况改善等目的。该学科的发展涉及机械、电子、通信、计算机等众多学科，其典型特点是涉及领域广、多学科交叉、与医学深度融合。因此，该学科的专业英语特点包括：

（1）长句多、被动句多、非谓语动词多、专业性强；

（2）由于学科不断交叉发展，产生了大量的复合词；

（3）随着技术的不断创新和发展，产生了大量的新词；

（4）为了行文简洁，应用大量的缩略词。

专业英语的词汇特点

生物医学工程学科的科技文章要求概念清晰，避免含糊不清和一词多义。为了准确、科学地表达观点，描述客观事实，遣词就显得尤为重要。该学科的专业英语最显著的特点体现在词汇的使用及构词法上。

1. 多用术语、专业性强

每个学科、行业或特定领域内都有其相应的专业术语，用于正确表达科学概念。专业术语与具体的科技领域息息相关，具有丰富的内涵和外延。生物医学工程领域也大量使用专业术语。例如，biomedical engineering（BME，生物医学工程）、magnetic resonance imaging（MRI，磁共振成像）、genetic engineering（基因工程）、active medical device（有源医疗器械）等都是专业性极强的词汇。此外，随着科技知识的普及，有些科技词汇已为大众所熟知，并演化为通用英语的一部分，如 cardiovascular disease（心血管疾病）、blood pressure（血压）等。

在科技文章中，词语的词义和专业紧密相关。如 device 一词，在通用英语中指"装置、器具、设备、仪器"；在生物医学工程领域常翻译成"器械"，如 active medical device（有源医疗器械）、non-active medical device（无源医疗器械）。对于这类词语，只有通过上下文和具体的语境才能确定其真正的含义。

2．大量源于希腊语或拉丁语

大量的科技词汇都源于希腊语或拉丁语，因为这两种语言的词义固定，概念清晰，也较少引起歧义。例如，一些来源于希腊语或拉丁语的名词在变复数时，遵循其源语言的变化规则，如 vertebra（椎骨）的复数形式是 vertebrae，thrombus（血栓）的复数形式是 thrombi，diagnosis（诊断）的复数形式是 diagnoses。再如，erythro-有 red 的意思，如 erythrocyte 意为红细胞；leuko-有 white 的意思，如 leukocyte 意为白细胞。下面列举一些源于希腊语或拉丁语的词缀或词根。

bio-	biotechnology 生物技术
derma-	dermatology 皮肤病学；dermatosis 皮肤病
homo-	homogenous 同质的，同类的
hydro-	hydrodynamic 流体的，水力的
mono-	monocyte 单核细胞
-cyte	monocyte 单核细胞；lymphocyte 淋巴细胞
-meter	thermometer 温度计；cytometer 血细胞计数器

3．新词不断、构词灵活

随着科技的日新月异，新事物、新概念和新现象的大量涌现，需要不断构造新的词汇。据统计，英语每年都能出现 5000 以上的新词汇。一般来说，科技英语新词汇的产生与其所属学科关系密切。生物医学工程领域产生的新词汇，包括 bioinformatics（生物信息学）、biophotonics（生物光子学）、biotechnology（生物技术）等。

为了更准确地表达这些新生事物，专业词汇的构词法也灵活多样，常见的构词法有词缀派生法、合成法、缩略法、混成法等。

1）词缀派生法

在英语中，常常在词根前、后分别加上前缀或后缀构成新词。通常来说，在构成新词的过程中，加前缀构成的新词只改变词义，词的属性一般不会改变。

本领域常用前缀举例如下。

（1）anti-/counter- 表示"反，抗"

anti-interference 抗干扰	antibody 抗体
antigen 抗原	antitoxin 抗毒素

counteraction 反作用   counterflow 反向流动

（2）auto- 表示"自动，自"

autocontrol 自控   automated 自动化的

（3）bio- 表示"生物的"

biomaterial 生物材料   biotechnology 生物技术

biocompatible 生物相容的   biomechanics 生物力学

（4）de- 表示"去，除"

defibrillator 除颤器   dehydration 脱水

（5）deci- 表示"十分之一"，常译为"分"

decibel (dB) 分贝   decimeter 分米   decimal 十进制的

（6）di- 表示"二"

dioxide 二氧化物   diode 二极管   dipole 偶极子

（7）electro- 表示"电的"

electrochemical 电化学的   electromagnetic 电磁的

（8）equi- 表示"同等，均"

equipartition 均分   equilibrium 均衡，平衡

（9）hydro- 表示"水"

hydrodynamic 流体的，水力的   hydroelectric 水力发电的

（10）hyper- 表示"高，超，重"

hypertension 高血压   hypersonic 高超声速的

（11）immuno- 表示"免疫，免疫的"

immunophenotyping 免疫表型   immunological 免疫学的

（12）inter- 表示"互相，（在）内，（在）中间"

interconnect 互连   interface 界面，接口

interchange 互换   interdisciplinary 跨学科的

（13）mega- 表示"兆，百万"

megawatt 兆瓦   megahertz 兆赫兹

（14）micro- 表示"微，百万分之一"

microwave 微波   microelectronics 微电子学

（15）mini- 表示"小"

minicomputer 小型计算机   minicell 微细胞

（16）neuro- 表示"神经的"

neuroengineering 神经工程   neuromuscular 神经肌肉的

（17）photo- 表示"光、光电，光敏"

photocell 光电池   photorectifier 光电检波器

（18）piezo- 表示"压"

  piezoelectric 压电的

（19）pre- 表示"在······前，预先"

  preheat 预热   preamplifier 前置放大器

（20）semi- 表示"半"

  semiconductor 半导体   semiautomatic 半自动的

（21）tele- 表示"远"

  telecontrol 遥控   telecommunications 电信

（22）thermo- 表示"热"

  thermoelectric 热电的   thermometer 温度计

（23）trans- 表示"转变，转换，变换，转移"

  transistor 晶体管   transplant 移植

（24）ultra- 表示"超"

  ultrasonic 超声的   ultraviolet 紫外线

  加后缀构成新词，主要改变词的属性。本领域常用后缀举例如下。

（1）-al（形容词词尾）

  digit 数字→digital 数字的 function 功能→functional 功能的

（2）-ance/-ence（名词词尾）

  capacitance 电容   resonance 谐振

（3）-en（动词词尾），一般是形容词+en，表示"使······"

  soft 软的→ soften 软化   short 短的→shorten 缩短

（4）-er/-or，表示"机器、设备、物件"等

  inductor 电感器   switcher 切换器

（5）-fold 接在数词后，构成形容词或副词，表示"······倍的"

  threefold 三倍的   thousandfold 一千倍的

（6）-free（形容词词尾），表示"无······的，免于······的"

  loss-free 无损耗的   oil-free 无油的

（7）-graphy（名词词尾），表示"图像制作技术"

  tomography 层析术   radiography 射线照相术

  mammography 乳房 X 射线照相术

（8）-ics（名词词尾）表示学科名称

  physics 物理学   electronics 电子学

（9）-let 表示"小"

  platelet 血小板   droplet 微滴

（10）-meter 表示"……表，……计"

　　ohmmeter 电阻表　　　　　　　　audiometer 听力计

（11）-metry（名词词尾）表示"测量法"

　　anthropometry 人体测量学　　　　cytometry 细胞计量术

　　photometry 测光　　　　　　　　morphometry 形态计量法

（12）-proof（形容词词尾）表示"防……的"

　　waterproof 防水的　　　　　　　lightning-proof 防雷的

（13）-scopy（名词词尾）表示"看或观察的行为"

　　uroscopy 尿检　　　　　　　　　fluoroscopy 荧光透视法

　　microscopy 显微镜检术　　　　　spectroscopy 光谱术

（14）-tion/-sion（名词词尾）

　　induce 感应→induction 感应　　　transmit 发射→transmission 传输，发射

（15）-type（名词词尾）表示"典型、范例、样板、类型"

　　prototype 原型、雏形　　　　　　phenotype（细胞的）表型

2）合成法

由两个或两个以上独立的词合在一起，构成一个新词。例如：

clean + room = cleanroom（洁净室）

pace + maker = pacemaker （起搏器）

light + weight = lightweight（轻量的、薄型的）

有的合成词的两个成分之间有连字符"-"。例如：

heat + resistant = heat-resistant（耐热的）

heart + lung machine = heart-lung machine（心肺机）

human + computer = human-computer （人机的）

专业英语中有很多专业术语由两个或更多的词组成，它们的构成成分虽然看起来是独立的，但实际上合起来才是一个完整的概念，因此也把它们看成一个术语。例如：

positron emission tomography（正电子发射断层显像术）

red blood cell（红细胞）

biomedical engineering（生物医学工程）

3）缩略法

将两个或多个单词进行省略或简化，组合成新词。可取多个词汇的首字母进行组合，或直接去掉词汇的某一部分。例如：

green fluorescence protein 缩略成 GFP（绿色荧光蛋白）

magnetic resonance image 缩略成 MRI（磁共振成像）

digital radiography 缩略成 DR（数字 X 射线摄影）

degree of freedom 缩略成 DOF（自由度）

photomultiplier tube 缩略成 PMT（光电倍增管）

computed tomography 缩略成 CT（计算机断层扫描术）

finite element analysis 缩略成 FEA（有限元分析）

range of motion 缩略成 ROM（关节活动度）

4）混成法

medical + care → medicare 医疗保健

positive + electron → positron 正电子

transfer + resistor → transistor 晶体管

专业英语的句法特点

1. 经常使用被动语态

被动语态在专业英语中用得非常频繁。首先，这是因为科技文章的主要目的是讲述客观现象，描写行为或状态本身，如介绍科技成果、仪器操作方法等，使用被动句比使用主动句主观色彩弱，能够突出论证主体本身。其次，行为或状态的主体有时没必要指出，或者根本指不出来。因此在专业英语中，凡是在不需要或不可能指出行为主体的场合，或者在需要突出行为客体的场合都使用被动语态。在很多情况下，被动结构也更简洁。例如：

（1）Flow cytometers are used in a range of applications from immunophenotyping, to ploidy analysis, to cell counting and green fluorescence protein (GFP) expression analysis.

参考译文：流式细胞仪在免疫分型、倍性分析、细胞计数和绿色荧光蛋白（GFP）表达分析等方面有广泛的应用。

（2）The signal-to-noise ration can be increased by changing a photomultiplier tube (PMT) gain directly instead of adjusting the gain of the preamplifier.

参考译文：信噪比不是通过调整前置放大器的增益，而是通过直接改变光电倍增管（PMT）的增益来提高的。

2. 多采用长难句

专业英语用于表达科学理论、技术原理、仪器维护方法等，常涉及各事物之间错综复杂的关系，而复杂的科学思维常无法用简单语句来表达，所以语法结构复杂的长句较多地应用于专业英语，而这种严谨周密、层次分明、重点突出的语言手段也就成为专业英语文体又一重要特征。为了保证表达内容的严密性、准确性和逻辑性，文中往往使用大量的复合句和有附加成分的长难句。一般来说，长难句的特点是后置定语、非谓语动词、宾语从句、状语从句等成分多。例如：

This view shows the primary systems of the flow cytometer schematically. These are: the fluidic system, which presents samples to the interrogation point and takes away the waste; the lasers, which are the light source for scatter and fluorescence; the optics, which gather and direct the light; the detectors, which receive the light; and, the electronics and the peripheral computer system, which convert the signals from the detectors into digital data and perform the necessary analyses.

3．大量使用名词化结构

名词化是指把动词通过加缀、转化等方式变成有动作含义的名词。专业英语要求行文简洁、表达客观、内容准确、信息量大，常强调存在的事实，而非某一行为，所以大量使用名称化结构。如果是动词短语或句子，则把其变成名词短语，例如：

（1）monitor heart diseases 可以转换成 monitoring of heart diseases。

（2）to examine specimens 可以转换成 the examination of specimens。

（3）biomedical engineers develop the equipment 可以转换成 the development of the equipment by biomedical engineers。

4．多用非谓语动词

每个简单的英文句子只能有一个谓语动词，作谓语的动词称为限定动词，不作谓语的动词或动词短语由于其结构不受主语的限定，没有人称和数的变化，因而称为非限定动词。非谓语动词（动词非限定形式）包括不定式（to + V）、V-ing 和过去分词（V-ed）。

1）非谓语动词不定式（to + V）

动词不定式短语在句中常用作主语、后置定语、表语、宾语、状语和宾语补足语。它们多以短语的形式出现，即以动词不定式为中心，再加上其他的状语、宾语。例如：

（1）The first step to solve the problem is to analyze the possible cause. （前者为后置定语，后者作表语）

（2）The electromotive force creates the electric pressure that causes the current to flow through a conductor. （作宾语补足语）

在专业英语中，不定式短语还常常单独放在句尾并用逗号隔开，用以补充说明作用或目的，或者放在句首并以逗号隔开，用以突出主句中所述事件的目的或作用。

（1）You need to find the regulation number that is the classification regulation for your device, to find the classification of your device, as well as whether any exemptions may exist.

（2）To find the classification of your device, as well as whether any exemptions may exist, you need to find the regulation number that is the classification regulation for your device.

2）非谓语动词 V-ing

在有的语法书中，V-ing 形式的动词分为动名词与现在分词，但现在常不加以区分。V-ing 在句中可作表语、主语、宾语、定语和宾语补足语等成分。由于该形式同时保留了动词性，因此可根据词性带上宾语或状语。例如：

（1）Physical, mental and emotional health is considered when treating a patient. （作状语）

（2）While taking up any home medical equipment, you need to take consultation from your doctor, nurses, or the specialist. （作状语）

（3）Having your blood pressure checked regularly indicates important fluctuations. （作主语）

在专业英语中，"with/without/for +（名词）+ V-ing"结构常用作补充说明。在这种结构中，with/without 没有词义，表示一种伴随情况，而 for 则多用于表示一些目的性动作，有时还用逗号隔开。例如：

（1）An MRI scan is the best way to see inside the human body, without cutting it open.

（2）As of 2009, the medical equipment industry is worth more than $200 billion globally, with the United States leading the market.

（3）An X-ray is very effective for showing doctors a broken bone.

3）非谓语动词 V-ed

由于动词的 V-ed 形式与 be 结合构成被动语态，与 have 连用构成完成时，因此，V-ed 形式本身含有被动与完成的意思。该形式在句中可作后置定语、状语等，保留了动词性，表示这一动作是已完成的或是被其修饰的名词（被动）接受的。V-ed 作定语常放在名词后面，含有被动的意思。例如：

（1）All metals are fairly hard, compared to polymers. （作状语）

（2）With an estimated 14 percent of the world's population expected to be 65 or older by 2030, the need for medical devices and qualified technicians to fix them will continue to grow. （作后置定语）

专业英语翻译技巧

通用英语翻译的要求是：信、达、雅。"信"是指忠实于原作的内容，翻译应尽可能地表达原文的意思。"达"是指翻译语言应流畅、易懂。在"信"的基础上，它进一步要求翻译通顺明白，并以接近母语的方式自然表达。"雅"则是指在翻译时选用的词语要得体，追求文章本身简明优雅。

专业英语翻译的要求则是：信、达、专业。

（1）信（faithful）：忠实，译文和原文是等义的，译文在内容上准确无误地传达原文的真实含义。

例句：This polymer material is not hard; it gives way to pressure.

初译：这个高分子材料不硬，它给压力让路（误译）。

改译：这个高分子材料不硬，受压就会变形。

（2）达（expressive）：流畅，通顺，符合中文的表达习惯，不能逐词死译。

例句：Measures have been taken to reduce risks of this medical device.

初译：一些措施已经被用来降低这个医疗器械的风险。

改译：目前已经采取了一些措施来降低这个医疗器械的风险。

（3）专业（professional）：科学性、严谨性，使用专业术语，不能说行外话。

例如，"Applied subfields of biomechanics include soft body dynamics, musculoskeletal & orthopedic biomechanics, animal locomotion & gait analysis, cardiovascular biomechanics, occupational biomechanics, rehabilitation, sports biomechanics, injury biomechanics, etc." 句中出现了较多的生物力学术语，在翻译时应注意使用符合译写规范的中文术语。

英、汉两种语言在语言结构与表达形式方面各有其自身的特点。专业英语中大量使用名词化结构、被动语态、复杂长句等，而汉语中动词、主动态和简单句用得多。此外，由于汉语中没有冠词、关系代词、关系副词、分词、不定式、动名词等词类或语言形式，因此，在专业英语翻译中，要使译文既忠实于原文又顺畅可读，就不能局限于逐词对等，必须采用适当的语态转换、句子成分顺序转换，以及句型转换等翻译技巧。

1. 根据专业领域确定词义

大量的词汇在专业英语中有其独特的词义，与其所属专业领域有关。同一个单词在不同的专业领域中可能具有完全不同的词义，即使在同一个领域中也可能有不同词义，举例如下。

（1）device：常译为"设备"，如"Operation of the device is extremely simple."可译为"该设备操作极为简单。"而在生物医学工程领域，常译为"器械"，如 medical device（医疗器械）。

（2）power：在数学中，常译为"幂"，如"The third power of two is 8."可译为"2 的 3 次幂为 8。"在电学中，常译为"电源、功率"，如 power meter（功率计）、electric power（电能）。

在阅读专业文献时，应注意扩大自己的专业词汇量，许多在通用英语中的单词，在专业领域也可能有其特定的词义。在确定词义时，可根据文章涉及的专业内容和上下文来确定。

2. 英语名词化结构及非谓语动词一般均可译成汉语的动词

专业英语中大量使用名词化结构，而汉语中则多使用动词，在翻译此类词组时可以予以转换处理，例句如下。

（1）A change of state from a solid to a liquid form requires heat energy.

参考译文：从固态变为液态需要热能。

（2）Light from the sun is a mixture of light of many different colors.

参考译文：太阳光是由许多不同颜色的光混合成的。

3. 被动语态用主动表达

专业英语往往强调如何去做，而不介意动作主体是谁，所以常采用被动语态。由于英语的许多被动句不需要或无法讲出动作的发出者，因此往往可译成汉语的无主句，而把原句中的主语译成宾语，例句如下。

（1）Now the heart can be safely opened and its valves can be repaired.

参考译文：现在可以安全地打开心脏，并对心脏瓣膜进行修复。

（2）Much progress has been made in biomedical engineering in less than a century.

参考译文：不到一个世纪，生物医学工程就取得了很大的进步。

（3）This medical device was formed from the same kind of materials that makes up that one.

参考译文：制造这个医疗器械的材料与制造那个医疗器械的材料是相同的。

当英语被动句中的主语为无生命的名词，且句中未出现由介词 by 引导的行为主体时，往往可译成汉语的主动句，原句的主语在译文中仍为主语。有时也可把原主语译成宾语，而把行为主体或相当于行为主体的介词宾语译成主语，例句如下。

（1）Materials may be grouped in several ways.

参考译文：材料可以按几种方式进行分组。

（2）In flow cytometry, sheath technique is used to make cells pass the interrogation point one at a time.

参考译文：在流式细胞术中，鞘流技术用来保证每次只有一个细胞通过检测点（激光照射区域）。

如果原句中未包含动作的发出者，在译成主动句时可以从逻辑主语出发，适当增添不确定主语，如"人们""大家""我们"等。凡是着重描述事物的过程、性质和状态的英语被动句，与系表结构相近，往往可以译成"是……"的结构。例句如下。

（1）Salt is known to have a very strong corroding effect on metals.

参考译文：大家知道，盐对金属有很强的腐蚀作用。

（2）Magnesium is found to be the best material for making flash light.

参考译文：人们发现，镁是制造闪光灯的最佳材料。

（3）The volume is not measured in square millimeters. It is measured in cubic millimeters.

参考译文：体积不是以平方毫米计量的，而是以立方毫米计量的。

（4）The first explosive in the world was made in China.

参考译文：世界上最早的炸药是在中国制造的。

4. 专业英语长难句翻译方法

专业英语长难句的结构特点是后置定语、非谓语动词、同位语、宾语从句、状语从句等修饰性成分多。这些成分相对复杂，既可以是单词、短语，也可以是从句，甚至有些句子能包含上述所有成分。一般情况下，简单句子中的某些主干成分（主语、谓语、宾语）会放在一起。长句表达虽然有条理性、周密性和严谨性，但是由于修饰性成分的大量存在，句中的主干成分常常被修饰性成分隔开，这就给翻译带来了很大困难。

值得注意的是，由于这些长难句通常都是由一些基本的句型扩展或变化而来，因此，翻译的关键在于抓住全句的主干成分，理解句子的中心意思。在此基础上，再去厘清句子的组织构成、成分间的连接关系，并补足附加成分的内容。一般来说，在翻译时可采用下列步骤：

① 厘清句子的逻辑关系，找出连接词汇；
② 辨别句子的主从结构，分切句子内容；
③ 省略句子的修饰性成分，找出句子的主干（主语、谓语、宾语）；
④ 根据上下文和全句内容领会句子的主要意思；
⑤ 根据上下层次和前后联系，补齐修饰性成分的内容。

例句如下。

（1）Most MRI systems use a superconducting magnet, which consists of many coils or windings of wire through which a current of electricity is passed, creating a magnetic field of up to 2.0 tesla.

参考译文：大多数的 MRI 系统使用超导磁体，它由许多线圈组成，线圈中有电流通过，可以产生一个 2.0 特斯拉的磁场。

（2）With an estimated 14 percent of the world's population expected to be 65 or older by 2030, the need for medical devices and qualified technicians to fix the will continue to grow.

参考译文：截至 2030 年，预计世界将有 14%的人口年龄在 65 岁以上，对于医疗器械及从事医疗器械维修的合格工程师的需求也将继续攀升。

（3）These measures are formulated according to the Law of the People's Republic of China on Import and Export Commodity Inspection (hereinafter referred to as the Inspection Law) and its implementing regulation and other relevant laws and administrative regulations for the purpose of strengthening the administration of inspection and supervision of the imported medical instruments and safeguarding the human health and life safety.

参考译文：为加强进口医疗器械检验监督管理，保障人体健康和生命安全，根据《中华人民共和国进出口商品检验法》（以下简称商检法）及其实施条例和其他有关法律法规规定，制定本办法。

Part I   General Descriptions on Biomedical Engineering

Unit 1   Introduction to Biomedical Engineering

In its broadest sense, biomedical engineering (BME) has been with us for centuries, perhaps even thousands of years. In 2000, German archeologists uncovered a 3,000-year-old mummy from Thebes with a wooden prosthetic tied to its foot to serve as a big toe. Researchers said the wear on the bottom surface suggests that it could be the oldest known limb prosthesis. Egyptians also used hollow reeds to look and listen to the internal goings-on of the human anatomy. In 1816, modesty prevented French physician Rene Laennec from placing his ear next to a young woman's bare chest, so he rolled up a newspaper and listened through it, triggering the idea for his invention that led to today's ubiquitous stethoscope.

In 1895, Wilhelm Roentgen (威廉・伦琴) accidentally discovered that a cathode-ray tube could make a sheet of paper coated with barium platinocyanide glow, even when the tube and the paper were in separate rooms. Roentgen decided the tube must be emitting some kind of penetrating rays, which he called "X" rays, indicating that they were an unknown form of radiation at the time. This set off a flurry of research into the tissue-penetrating and tissue-destroying properties of X-rays, a line of research that ultimately produced the modern array of medical imaging technologies and virtually eliminated the need for exploratory surgery. Ever since then, biomedical engineering has developed rapidly and obtained excellent achievements.

During the second half of the 20th century, major upgrades were seen in medical devices. One of the very first experiments conducted was by Willem Kolff (威廉・考尔夫), who was known as the pioneer for modern dialysis. He was an inventor, doctor, and researcher. He was a firm believer in the fact that advancing technologies could be used to treat diseases. Being one of the lead designers of the first mechanical heart which could be implanted and the inventor of what is now known as the heart-lung machine which made open-heart surgery attainable, he was the receiver of many awards including Albert Lasker

Award for Clinical Medical Research (艾伯特 · 拉斯克临床医学研究奖). By the 1960s, biomedical engineering departments were formed at many prestigious universities including Duke University, Johns Hopkins University, Case Western Reserve University, and the University of Virginia, all of which remain an integral part of cutting-edge research on BME that goes on.

Biomedical engineering is the application of engineering principles and design concepts to medicine and biology for health care purposes (e.g. diagnostic or therapeutic). This field seeks to close the gap between engineering and medicine, combining the design and problem-solving skills of engineering with medical and biological sciences to advance health care treatment, including diagnosis, monitoring, and therapy. Biomedical engineering has only recently emerged as its own study, compared to many other engineering fields. Such an evolution is common as a new field transition from being an interdisciplinary specialization among already-established fields, to being considered a field in itself. Much of the work in biomedical engineering consists of research and development, spanning a broad array of subfields. Prominent biomedical engineering applications include the development of biocompatible prostheses, various diagnostic and therapeutic medical devices ranging from clinical equipment to micro-implants, common imaging equipment such as MRIs and EEGs, regenerative tissue growth, pharmaceutical drugs, and therapeutic biologicals.

Biomedical engineering involves applying the concepts, knowledge, and approaches of virtually all engineering disciplines (e.g. electrical, mechanical, and chemical engineering, etc.) to solve specific health care related problems. It is thus an interdisciplinary branch of engineering encompassing bioinformatics, biomaterial, tissue engineering, etc. Fig 1.1 shows the typical branches of biomedical engineering.

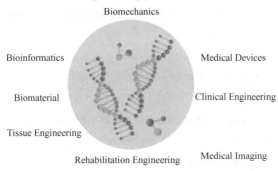

Fig 1.1   Typical branches of biomedical engineering

1.1   Bioinformatics

Bioinformatics is an interdisciplinary field that develops methods and software tools for understanding biological data. As an interdisciplinary field of science, bioinformatics combines computer science, statistics, mathematics, and engineering to analyze and interpret biological data.

Nowadays, bioinformatics also combines computer programming, big data, and biology to help scientists understand and identify patterns in biological data. It is particularly useful in studying genomes and DNA sequencing, as it allows scientists to organize large amounts of data.

1.2　Biomaterial

A biomaterial is any matter, surface, or construct that interacts with living systems. The study of biomaterials is called biomaterials science or biomaterials engineering. Biomaterials play an integral role in medicine today — restoring function and facilitating healing for people after injury or disease. They may be natural or synthetic and are used in medical applications to support, enhance, or replace damaged tissue or a biological function. It has experienced steady and strong growth over its history, with many companies investing large amounts of money into the development of new products. It encompasses elements of medicine, biology, chemistry, tissue engineering and material science.

Metals, ceramics, plastic, glass, and even living cells and tissues all can be used in creating a biomaterial. They can be reengineered into molded or machined parts, coatings, fibers, films, foams, and fabrics for use in biomedical products and devices. These may include heart valves, hip joint replacements, dental implants, or contact lenses. They often are biodegradable, and some are bio-absorbable, meaning they are eliminated gradually from the body after fulfilling a function.

1.3　Tissue Engineering

Tissue engineering, like genetic engineering, is a major segment of biotechnology — which overlaps significantly with BME. One of the goals of tissue engineering is to create artificial organs (via biological material) for patients that need organ transplants. Biomedical engineers are currently researching methods of creating such organs. Researchers have grown solid jawbones and tracheas from human stem cells towards this end. Several artificial urinary bladders have been grown in laboratories and transplanted successfully into human patients.

1.4   Medical Devices

This is an extremely broad category — essentially covering all health care products that do not achieve their intended results through predominantly chemical (e.g. pharmaceuticals) or biological (e.g. vaccines) means, and do not involve metabolism.

A medical device is intended for use in,

- the diagnosis of disease or other conditions, or
- in the cure, mitigation, treatment, or prevention of disease.

Some examples include pacemakers, infusion pumps, heart-lung machines, dialysis machines, artificial organs, implants, artificial limbs, corrective lenses, cochlear implants, ocular prosthetics, facial prosthetics, and dental implants.

1.5   Medical Imaging

Medical/biomedical imaging is a major segment of medical devices. This area deals with enabling clinicians to directly or indirectly "view" things not visible in plain sight (such as due to their size, and/or location). This can involve utilizing ultrasound, magnetism, ultra-violet, radiology, and other means.

Imaging technologies are often essential to medical diagnosis, and are typically the most complex equipment found in a hospital, including fluoroscopy, magnetic resonance imaging (MRI), nuclear medicine, positron emission tomography (PET), PET-CT scans, projection radiography such as X-rays and CT scans, tomography, ultrasound, optical microscopy, and electron microscopy.

1.6   Clinical Engineering

Clinical engineering is the branch of biomedical engineering dealing with the actual implementation of medical equipment and technologies in hospitals or other clinical settings. Major roles of clinical engineers include training and supervising biomedical equipment technicians, selecting technological products/services and managing their implementation, working with governmental regulators on inspections/audits, and serving as technological consultants for other hospital staff (e.g. physicians, administrators, I.T., etc.). Clinical engineers also advise and collaborate with medical device producers regarding prospective design improvements based on clinical experiences, as well as monitoring the progression of the state-of-the-art so as to redirect procurement patterns accordingly.

1.7　Rehabilitation Engineering

Rehabilitation engineering is the systematic application of engineering sciences to design, develop, adapt, test, evaluate, apply, and distribute technological solutions to problems confronted by individuals with disabilities. Functional areas addressed through rehabilitation engineering may include mobility, communications, hearing, vision, and cognition, and activities associated with employment, independent living, education, and integration into the community.

The rehabilitation process for people with disabilities often entails the design of assistive devices such as walking aids intended to promote inclusion of their users into the mainstream of society, commerce, and recreation.

1.8　Biomechanics

Biomechanics is closely related to engineering, because it often uses traditional engineering sciences to analyze biological systems. Some simple applications of Newtonian mechanics and/or materials sciences can supply correct approximations to the mechanics of many biological systems. Applied mechanics, most notably mechanical engineering disciplines such as continuum mechanics, mechanism analysis, structural analysis, kinematics and dynamics play prominent roles in the study of biomechanics.

Usually, biological systems are much more complex than man-built systems. Numerical methods are hence applied in almost every biomechanical study. Research is done in an iterative process of hypothesis and verification, including several steps of modeling, computer simulation and experimental measurements.

Applied subfields of biomechanics include soft body dynamics, animal locomotion & gait analysis, musculoskeletal & orthopedic biomechanics, occupational biomechanics, cardiovascular biomechanics, rehabilitation, sports biomechanics, injury biomechanics, etc.

Words and Expressions

biomedical engineering (BME)	生物医学工程
implant ['ɪmplɑːnt]	*n.* （植入人体中的）移植物，植入物
heart-lung machine	心肺机
therapeutic [ˌθerə'pjuːtɪk]	*adj.* 治疗的，医疗的，治病的
interdisciplinary [ˌɪntəˌdɪsə'plɪnəri]	*adj.* 多学科的，跨学科的

biocompatible [ˌbaɪəʊkəm'pætɪbl]   *adj.* 生物相容的

prosthesis [prɒs'θiːsɪs]   *n.* 假体

electroencephalography [ɪˌlektrəʊm'sefələɡrɑːfi](EEG)   *n.* 脑电图

bioinformatics [ˌbaɪəʊɪnfə'mætɪks]   *n.* 生物信息学

biomaterial ['baɪəʊməˌtɪəriəl]   *n.* 生物材料，生物材料学

tissue engineering   组织工程

DNA sequencing   DNA 测序

genetic engineering   基因工程

artificial organ   人工器官

stem cell   干细胞

pacemaker ['peɪsˌmeɪkə]   *n.* 起搏器

infusion pump   输液泵

artificial limb   假肢

dialysis machine   透析机

corrective lenses   矫正眼镜，矫正镜片

cochlear implant   人工耳蜗

ocular prosthetics   眼修复术

facial prosthetics   面部修复术

dental implant   牙科植入体

fluoroscopy [flʊə'rɒskəpɪ]   *n.* 荧光学，荧光透视法

magnetic resonance imaging (MRI)   磁共振成像

nuclear medicine   核医学

positron emission tomography (PET)   正电子发射断层显像

PET-CT scan   PET-CT 扫描

projection radiography   放射照相术

X-ray   X 射线

CT scan   CT 扫描

tomography [tə'mɒɡrəfi]   *n.* 层析术，层析成像

ultrasound ['ʌltrəsaʊnd]   *n.* 超声波，超声，超声波扫描检查

optical microscopy   光学显微术

electron microscopy   电子显微镜术，电子显微术

clinical engineering   临床工程

rehabilitation [ˌriːhəbɪlɪ'teɪʃən]   *n.* 康复

rehabilitation engineering   康复工程

biomechanics [ˌbaɪəʊmə'kænɪks]   *n.* 生物力学

continuum mechanics   连续介质力学

mechanism analysis	机构分析
structural analysis	结构分析
kinematics [ˌkɪnɪ'mætɪks]	n. 运动学
dynamics [daɪ'næmɪks]	n. 动力学
gait analysis	步态分析
musculoskeletal & orthopedic biomechanics	肌肉骨骼与骨科生物力学
occupational biomechanics	职业生物力学
cardiovascular biomechanics	心血管生物力学
sports biomechanics	运动生物力学
injury biomechanics	损伤生物力学
technical term	技术术语，专业术语

Key Sentences

1. Biomedical engineering is the application of engineering principles and design concepts to medicine and biology for health care purposes (e.g. diagnostic or therapeutic). This field seeks to close the gap between engineering and medicine, combining the design and problem-solving skills of engineering with medical and biological sciences to advance health care treatment, including diagnosis, monitoring, and therapy.

参考译文： 生物医学工程是将工程原理和设计概念应用于医学和生物学，以达到医疗健康目的（如诊断或治疗）的学科领域。该领域旨在弥合工程学和医学之间的差距，将工程学的设计方法和解决问题的技能与医学、生物科学相结合，以推进包括诊断、监测治疗在内的医疗保健事业的发展。

2. Biomedical engineering has only recently emerged as its own study, compared to many other engineering fields. Such an evolution is common as a new field transition from being an interdisciplinary specialization among already-established fields, to being considered a field in itself.

参考译文： 与许多其他工程领域相比，生物医学工程近年来才作为一门（学科）研究出现。从原有领域中的跨学科专业发展为一门独立学科，这种演变是常见的。

3. Biomedical engineering involves applying the concepts, knowledge, and approaches of virtually all engineering disciplines (e.g. electrical, mechanical, and chemical engineering, etc.) to solve specific health care related problems. It is thus an interdisciplinary branch of engineering encompassing bioinformatics, biomaterial, tissue engineering, etc.

参考译文： 生物医学工程几乎涉及所有工程学科领域（如电气、机械和化学工程等），致力于应用相关概念、知识和方法来解决特定的医疗健康问题。因此，它是一个具有跨学科属性的工程学分支，包括生物信息学、生物材料和组织工程等细分领域。

Further Readings

Biomedical Engineering: Its Introduction and Sub-Disciplinary Fields

Biomedical (related to the activities and applications of science to clinical medicine) engineering is the use of engineering principles and methods to the medical field. The convention of this field is to overcome the breach between medicine and engineering. For the improvement of health care monitoring, therapy and diagnosis, biomedical engineering combines the design and problem-solving abilities of engineering with biological and medical sciences.

Biomedical engineering is basically about research and development. It crosses a broad range of subfields. These sub-disciplinary fields are listed as follows.

- **Biomechanics**. It is the branch of biophysics that deals with the mechanics of the human or animal body. It especially concerns with muscles and skeleton or the functioning of a particular part of a body.

- **Biomaterials**. It is any matter, surface, or construct that interacts with biological systems.

- **Bio-mechatronics**. It is an applied interdisciplinary science that aims to integrate mechanical elements, electronics and parts of biological organisms.

- **Bionics**. It is also known as biomimicry, biomimetics, or bioinspiration. It is the application of biological methods and systems found in nature to the study and design of engineering systems and modern technology.

- **Clinical engineering**. It is a specialty of biomedical engineering responsible primarily for applying and implementing medical technology to optimize health care delivery.

- **Bioinstrumentation**. It is the application of electronics and measurement principles and techniques to develop devices used in diagnosis and treatment of disease.

- **Bio-nanotechnology**. It usually refers to the intersection of biotechnology and nanotechnology.

- **Medical imaging**. It is the technique and process used to create images of the human body (or parts and function thereof) for clinical purposes (medical procedures seeking to reveal, diagnose or examine disease) or medical science including the study of normal anatomy and physiology.

- **Cellular engineering**. It is a new field that addresses issues related to understanding and manipulating cell structure-function relationships.

- **Tissue engineering**. It is a subfield of biomaterials, which is the use of a combination of cells, engineering and materials methods, and suitable biochemical and physiochemical factors to improve or replace biological functions.

- **Genetic engineering or genetic modification**. It is the direct human manipulation of an organism's material in a way that does not occur under natural conditions. It involves the use of recombinant DNA techniques, but does not include traditional animal and plant breeding or mutagenesis.

- **Neural engineering or neuro-engineering**. It is a discipline within biomedical engineering that uses engineering techniques to understand, repair, replace, enhance, or otherwise exploit the properties of neural systems.

- **Pharmaceutical engineering**. It is a branch of pharmaceutical technology that involves development, commercialization and manufacturing components within the pharmaceuticals industry.

- **System physiology**. It is the science of the mechanical, physical, bioelectrical, and biochemical functions of humans in good health, studying their organs, and the cells of which they are composed. Physiology focuses principally on the level of organs and systems.

- **Rehabilitation engineering**. It is the systematic application of engineering sciences to design, develop, adapt, test, evaluate, apply, and distribute technological solutions to problems confronted by individuals with disabilities.

Biomedical Engineering and Biomedical Engineers

No matter what the date is, biomedical engineering has provided advances in medical technology to improve human health. Biomedical engineering achievements range from early devices, such as crutches, platform shoes, wooden teeth, and the ever-changing cache of instruments in a doctor's black bag, to more modern marvels, including pacemakers, the heart-lung machine, dialysis machines, diagnostic equipment, imaging technologies of every kind, and artificial organs, implants and advanced prosthetics. It is estimated that about thirty thousand biomedical engineers are working in various areas of health technology.

A biomedical engineer uses traditional engineering expertise to analyze and solve problems in biology and medicine, providing an overall enhancement of health care. Students choose the biomedical engineering field to be of service to people, to partake of the excitement of working with living systems, and to apply advanced technology to the complex problems of medical care. The biomedical engineer works with other health care professionals including physicians, nurses, therapists and technicians. Biomedical engineers may be called upon in a wide range of capacities: to design instruments, devices, and software, to bring together knowledge from many technical sources to develop new procedures, or to conduct research needed to solve clinical problems.

Top Schools for Biomedical Engineering in the USA

Biomedical engineering is a growing field that is projected to keep expanding as populations increase in both number and age. For this reason, more and more schools have been adding biomedical engineering to their STEM (i.e. sciences, technological fields, engineering disciplines, and mathematics) offerings. The best schools for biomedical engineering tend to have large programs with a talented faculty, well-equipped research facilities, and access to area hospitals and medical facilities.

Duke University. Duke's BME department is just a short walk from the highly regarded Duke University Hospital and School of Medicine, so it has been easy to develop meaningful collaborations between engineering and the health sciences. The program is supported by 45 tenured or tenure-track faculty members and graduates more than 100 bachelor's degree students a year. Duke is home to 10 centers and institutes related to biomedical engineering.

Georgia Institute of Technology. Georgia Institute of Technology is one of the nation's top public universities, and it tends to rank highly for all engineering fields. Biomedical engineering is no exception. The university's Atlanta location is a true asset, and the BME program has a strong research and educational partnership with neighboring Emory University. The program emphasizes problem-based learning, design, and independent research, so students graduate with plenty of hands-on experience.

Johns Hopkins University. Johns Hopkins does not typically top the lists of best engineering programs, but biomedical engineering is a clear exception. Johns Hopkins often ranks first in the country for BME. The university has long been a leader in biological and health sciences from the undergraduate to doctoral levels. Research opportunities abound with 10 affiliated centers and institutes, and the university is proud of its new BME Design Studio—an open floor-plan workspace where students can meet, brainstorm, and create prototypes of biomedical devices.

Massachusetts Institute of Technology(MIT). MIT graduates about 50 biomedical engineers each year, and another 50 from its BME graduate programs. The institute has long had a well-funded program for supporting and encouraging undergraduate research, and undergraduate students can work alongside graduate students, faculty members, and medical professionals at the school's 10 affiliated research centers.

Stanford University. The three pillars of Stanford's Basic Science and Engineering (BSE) program — Measure, Model, Make — highlight the school's emphasis on the act of creating. The program resides jointly in the School of Engineering and the School of Medicine leading to unimpeded collaboration between engineering and the life sciences.

Stanford has the facilities and resources to support a wide range of biomedical engineering research.

Top Schools for Biomedical Engineering in China

BME in Shanghai Jiao Tong University (SJTU)

The Biomedical Engineering (BME) program was founded in 1979, among the first established ones in China. Since its establishment, it has been consistently ranked among the top three in China by the Ministry of Education, based on national assessment conducted every five years. The School of BME at SJTU was established in 2011. Since its establishment, the school has aimed at excellence in both teaching and research for developing advanced medical technologies with contribution to human health and unmet clinical needs. It has placed a particular emphasis on "interdisciplinary, international collaboration, and concrete clinical applications". Currently, the program has three main research themes: 1) biomedical instrumentation; 2) nano, molecular and regenerative medicine; and 3) imaging, computational and systems biomedicine. To nurture the next generation leaders in BME, the program has focused on the ability of the students to master and synthesize knowledge across different disciplines with in-depth understanding of the human and societal needs from different cultures and economic backgrounds.

BME in Tsinghua University

It is one of the first universities that established the interdisciplinary biomedical engineering, and the Department of Biomedical Engineering remains in top ranking in China. Under the mentorship of China's leading researchers and engineers, students will apply engineering principles to answer important biomedical problems and translate their findings into new applications. Research fields include biomedical data science, biomedical imaging & instrumentation, computational medicine, genomics and systems biology, neuro-engineering, and regenerative and immune engineering.

BME in Zhejiang University

It is one of the important bases of China for cultivating senior talents in biomedical engineering and instrument science. It has good conditions for scientific research and education. It has a number of key laboratories, such as Biomedical Transducer National Special Lab and Key Laboratory of Biomedical Engineering, Ministry of Education.

The researches here have been focused on biomedical information, biomedical sensor and detection, quantitative & systemic physiology and neural engineering, medical image and image signal processing, biomaterials and cell engineering and biophotonics.

BME in University of Shanghai for Science and Technology

Biomedical engineering is a highly interdisciplinary emerging discipline among already-established subjects including science, engineering, medicine, biology etc. With the continuing high-technology development and increasing medical needs, researches in biomedical engineering have been expanded from medical electronics and medical imaging, to biomaterials, tissue engineering, medical instrument and bioinformatics etc.

With strong academic focus on engineering, University of Shanghai for Science and Technology attaches great significance to research and development (R&D), design and manufacturing. Under such a background, biomedical engineering places equal emphasis on both theoretical and applied research closely related to medical instrument, a key area with national key support through critical technological breakthroughs, research-based development of new medical instrument as well as the cultivation of creative talents with the goal of better serving medical device industry and benefiting the whole society.

Based on medical device industry, the discipline of biomedical engineering has witnessed the progress of diverse researches with engineering characteristics conducted in the fields of micro-invasive medical instrument, cryogenic biomedical engineering, which take the lead in China, rehabilitation engineering, medical informatics and so on.

Micro-invasive medical instrument and technology, with key issues and technology in interventional micro-invasive medical instrument and micro-invasive surgical instruments as its major research field, is committed to the research and development of products of independent intellectual property rights, filling the gaps in the field in China. More than 100 products such as interventional medical instrument and implantable medical instrument have been developed since the Engineering Research Center for Modern Micro-invasive Medical Instrument and Technology was approved by the Ministry of Education after being co-applied by University of Shanghai for Science and Technology and Micro-port Medical Company (Shanghai).

Cryo-biomedical engineering has been on a leading position in China, with its research mainly covering bio-thermal science such as cells, tissues and even the entire human body since it was established 30 years ago. In collaboration with more than a dozen hospitals, the concentration introduced or improved theoretical and technical methods in cryogenic storage and freeze-drying, developed a wide range of cryogenic biomedical equipment such as cryoprobe, cooling device, cryogenic storage instrument, and successfully achieved cryopreservation or freeze-drying for living cells and tissues, providing support for clinical services, such as cryopreservation of skin, pancreatic islet cells, trachea and arteries. Biomedical information and processing covers fundamental studies in pathogenesis of major human diseases, biological genomics and health informatics, the outcomes of which include research on pathogenesis of major human diseases from molecular and genetic perspectives, acquisition and analysis of medical imaging, and development of high-frequency ultrasound microscope, digital medical instrument as well as computer-aided detection and diagnosis (CAD) technology on the basis of medical imaging.

Unit 2　Differences Between Bioengineering and Biomedical Engineering

Bioengineering and biomedical engineering are highly interdisciplinary branches of study. These specializations can be twisted together, but their scope and applications differ considerably. Though they are related with each other, students must understand and compare them very carefully before opting for a career depending upon their areas of interest.

Bioengineering focuses on the application of engineering on biological processes, food, agriculture and environmental processes. On the other hand, biomedical engineering focuses on the application of engineering to biological and medical sciences to improve health care delivery systems.

2.1　Research Areas

Bioengineering, also called biological engineering, is the study of applied engineering practices in general biology. It is the broader topic when compared to biomedical engineering. Bioengineering covers topics such as agriculture, pharmaceuticals, natural resources and foodstuffs, etc. In addition, it covers general medical practices, though biomedical engineering focuses more on this field than general bioengineering does. Bioengineering practices are applied to many different industries, including health care, but biological engineering practices are not explicitly for medical purposes.

Biomedical engineering is a more specialized version of bioengineering, utilizing many of the discipline's principal theories and putting them to practice to improve human health. The field is focused on the production of new tools and processes that can be used in various health care contexts. Of all the fields of engineering, a biomedical engineer is likely to have one of the largest impacts on a person's life. Biomedical engineers commonly work to solve issues that are present in the life sciences; those that work on prosthetics or the emerging field of cybernetics (more formally known as biomechatronics) may also be referred to as biomechanical engineers. Items like the pacemaker, artificial heart and cochlear implant are all results of biomedical innovation. Medical and surgical tools such as specialized robotic surgery suites also fall under their purview, or to be more specific, the category of medical device engineering. Biomedical engineers also work to advance the efficacy of natural processes through biotechnology, such as tissue regeneration and cell diffusion. These engineers can be found in almost all fields of medicine. Wherever there's a problem, they work to find a solution.

The main difference between bioengineering and biomedical engineering is that bioengineering theoretically focuses on different areas of natural science to solve several issues; on the other hand, biomedical engineering focuses practically in the context of health. Biomedical engineering is said to be a more specialized version of bioengineering.

Biomedical engineering is the application of engineering tools for solving problems in biology and medicine. It is an engineering discipline that is practiced by professionals trained primarily as engineers, but with a specialized focus on the medical and biological applications of classical engineering principles. Fig 2.1 shows the relationship between biology, medicine and engineering.

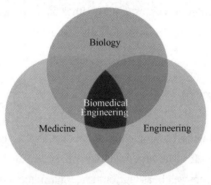

Fig 2.1　Relationship between biology, medicine and engineering

2.2　Education and Personal Needs

Both prospective bioengineers and biomedical engineers need a certain set of similar skills in order to thrive in these fields. Since much of the work involves synthesizing solutions to complex problems, applicants should have strong problem-solving skills and the perseverance necessary to see tough projects through to the end. A desire to confront challenge is a great trait to have for anyone looking to enter engineering disciplines, and this goes double for the biological disciplines. A grasp of the scientific method and the associated discipline it requires is a necessity, and those with analytical minds are best suited to these roles. Indecisiveness can be a major weakness to those who otherwise might fit the biological sciences well— while decisions are not usually made under the pressure of time like they would be for practitioners of medicine, the impact of choice is long-lasting in any engineering discipline. If you are confident in your decision-making ability and possess the aforementioned skills, then biomedical and biological engineering would be great fits for you.

The coursework for each degree is fairly similar. A basic engineering curriculum defines both bioengineering and biomedical engineering at most institutions, as the application of engineering principles is just as important in biological sciences as it is in other fields. Mathematics is another universal foundational skill: calculus, differential equations, and advanced statistics are necessary skills in both degree programs. Advanced knowledge of biology is another part of these curricula, and physics, chemistry and other sciences get a fair amount of focus as well. At the conclusion of a degree program, many colleges have students conduct capstone projects, where their engineering skills will be applied to create prototype products or processes that solve specific issues in biological scientific fields.

2.3   Job Duties

General bioengineering and biomedical engineering jobs can be found in many different fields. Bioengineers can find work in agriculture, health care, pharmaceuticals, food and drink production, and many more industries. Biomedical engineers also have a breadth of job possibilities at their disposal despite their narrower focus, as practically every field of medicine makes use of biomedical engineers. Medical technology engineering roles are also available, along with specialized positions in areas such as bioinstrumentation, medical imaging and even genetic engineering.

Medical device engineers design and develop medical-technical systems, installations, and equipment such as pacemakers, MRI scanners, and X-ray machines. They monitor the whole manufacturing process from concept design to product implementation. Activities undertaken include, among others, designing product improvements, developing methods and techniques to evaluate design suitability, coordinating initial production, developing test procedures, and designing manufacturing diagrams.

2.4   Job Outlook

Both careers of bioengineering and biomedical engineering have strong job security and are parts of growing industries. However, the presence of technology in the medical field is growing every day. Biomedical engineers can contribute in many different ways to this growing need. Engineers can create new types of software to assist medical professionals in diagnosing ailments and managing health care records. They can develop new medical devices to make procedures such as spinal taps or blood samples quick and painless for patients. And they can even invent new biological materials that assist in digestion and contribute to healthy gut flora. Despite the specific focus of biomedical engineers when compared to bioengineers, the possibilities are just as exciting.

Bioengineers and biomedical engineers can expect to receive excellent benefits, as most technology and engineering professionals can. Graduates can expect vacation and paternity leave, paid time off, paid sick time, and medical insurance. As you advance in your career, additional opportunities will open to you. Dental, vision and pet insurance can be at your disposal, as can remote work arrangements, depending on your job.

Words and Expressions

agriculture ['ægrɪˌkʌltʃə]	*n.* 农业
pharmaceuticals [ˌfɑːmə'sjuːtɪkəlz]	*n.* 药物
foodstuff ['fuːdstʌf]	*n.* 食物，食品
cybernetics [ˌsaɪbə'netɪks]	*n.* 控制论
biomechatronics [baɪəʊˌmekə'trɒnɪks]	*n.* 生物机械电子学
artificial heart	人工心脏
robotic surgery suites	机器人手术套件
tissue regeneration	组织再生
cell diffusion	细胞扩散
capstone project	顶点课程，高级论文或高级研讨会
prototype ['prəʊtətaɪp]	*n.* 原型
bioinstrumentation [baɪəʊˌɪnstrʊmen'teɪʃn]	*n.* 生物仪器
ailment ['eɪlmənt]	*n.* 小病，轻病
spinal tap	腰椎穿刺
gut flora	肠道菌群

Key Sentences

1. Biomedical engineering is a more specialized version of bioengineering, utilizing many of the discipline's principal theories and putting them to practice to improve human health.

参考译文：生物医学工程是生物工程的一个更细分的专业，它利用了该学科的许多重要理论，并将其付诸实践，以改善人类的健康状况。

2. A desire to confront challenge is a great trait to have for anyone looking to enter engineering disciplines, and this goes double for the biological disciplines.

参考译文：乐于直面挑战对于任何想进入工程学科的人来说都是一种很好的特质，而这一点对于生物学科来说加倍有益。

3. Activities undertaken include, among others, designing product improvements, developing methods and techniques to evaluate design suitability, coordinating initial production, developing test procedures, and designing manufacturing diagrams.

参考译文：除此之外，开展的活动还包括设计产品改进、开发用于评估设计适用性的方法和技术、协调初始生产、开发测试程序和设计制造图。

Further Readings

What Is Bioengineering?

Bioengineering or biological engineering is a course that deals theoretically with life sciences, physical sciences, engineering principles, mathematics, and problem-solving in biology, health, medicines, and other fields.

In simple words, bioengineering can be defined as the applied engineering practices in general biology. It is a vast field that even covers agriculture, pharmaceuticals, topics related to food, natural resources, etc.

Bioengineering covers several aspects of traditional engineering fields, including chemical, electrical, mechanical engineering, etc. A bioengineering graduate can be employed in several institutions as they know medical devices, pharmaceuticals, etc. They can even pursue careers in law, business, or any other field of their choice.

Few examples that bioengineering covers are: medical image techniques including MRI or X-ray, the study of artificial organs like an artificial hip, joints, knees etc., and using engineering principles in fields of pharmaceuticals for manufacturing purposes.

The complexity of the course makes it vast, and thus preferred by fewer people. The specialized courses within bioengineering like biomedical engineering are preferred more due to the clarity of field it offers. Bioengineering mostly offers research work as the discipline covers the theory part more.

What Is Biomedical Engineering?

Biomedical engineering is a more specialized version of bioengineering, which uses several theories of different disciplines' principles and utilizes them practically to improve human health. This field of engineering is more focused on developing tools and techniques within the medical devices and human health care context.

In other words, biomedical engineering for biomedical engineers deals with diagnosis, therapy and monitoring. Biomedical engineers have the scope in several fields related to medical and health care.

Biomedical engineering is now evolving as an entirely different field which is itself a disciplinary course instead of an interdisciplinary course. Now it offers several interdisciplinary courses such as biomechanics, tissue engineering, biomedical optics, bioinformatics, biomaterials, pharmaceutical engineering, neural engineering and so on.

Biomedical engineers can also go for research work, or simply be hired as biomedical equipment technicians (BMET) in any hospital, who work for routine maintenance of devices. They usually have an innovative job for solving medical issues, like the invention of artificial hearts, artificial joints, regeneration of tissues, etc.

Biomedical engineering is great scope for people who want to go for research work in health care context but do not want to perform a surgery. This disciplinary course offers the research work and even the practical knowledge about engineering principles of several other disciplinary courses of bioengineering.

Main Differences Between Bioengineering and Biomedical Engineering

(1) Bioengineering is a course that deals theoretically with life sciences, physical sciences, engineering principles, mathematics, and problem-solving in biology, health, medicines, and other fields, whereas biomedical engineering is a specialized version of bioengineering.

(2) Bioengineering is a theory-based disciplinary course. On the other hand, biomedical engineering is a more practical knowledge-based course.

(3) Bioengineering is a vast field that covers several other interdisciplinary courses including biomedical engineering. On the other hand, biomedical engineering is itself a specialized course of bioengineering.

(4) Bioengineering does not necessarily deal with health and care. On the other hand, biomedical engineering deals with health and care.

(5) Biomedical engineering is a more preferred course as compared to bioengineering.

(6) Bioengineering is a broad disciplinary course that covers several other fields like agriculture, natural resources, etc., but biomedical engineering explicitly works within the boundaries of health and care.

Table 2.1 shows the comparison between bioengineering and biomedical engineering.

Table 2.1   Comparison between bioengineering and biomedical engineering

Items	Bioengineering	Biomedical Engineering
Definition	It deals theoretically with life sciences, physical sciences, engineering principles, mathematics, and problem-solving in biology, health, medicines, and other fields	It is a more specialized version of bioengineering, which uses several theories of different disciplines' principles and utilizes them practically to improve human health
Other inclusive courses	Biomedical engineering, etc.	Bioinformatics, neural engineering, etc.
Type of knowledge	Theory	Practical
Fields	Agriculture, natural resources, health, etc.	Health and care
Popularity level	Less preferred	More preferred

Top Schools in the USA

Bioengineering and biomedical engineering are not always offered at the same school. Table 2.2 shows a list of schools in the USA that offer bioengineering and biomedical engineering as majors.

Table 2.2   Top schools offering BE and BME in the USA

Schools Offering Bioengineering	Schools Offering Biomedical Engineering
California Institute of Technology	Arizona State University
San Diego State University	California Polytechnic State University
Stanford University	Colorado State University
University of California, Berkeley	Yale University
University of California, Los Angeles	George Washington University
University of Hawaii at Manoa	University of Florida
Syracuse University	Northwestern University
Oregon State University	Purdue University
University of Pennsylvania	Tulane University
Rice University	Johns Hopkins University
University of Washington	Boston University

Unit 3 Biomedical Sensors and Biomedical Instrumentation

3.1 Definition of a Sensor

Sensors are everywhere, be it whether we are engineers, doctors or anyone, we are surrounded by sensors. It is a device that converts signals from one energy domain to electrical domain which you commonly see in your homes, offices, shopping malls, hospitals, like fire sensors and door sensors which makes our life easier and safer.

There is no uniform definition of exactly what a sensor or transducer is. In general, a sensor is usually defined as a device that detects a condition and generates an optical, electrical, chemical, or mechanical signal. A transducer is a device that converts energy from one form to another and forms part of the sensor. Sensors are critical components in all devices and measurement systems.

3.2 Classifying Sensors

Classifying sensors is not an easy task. Classification may be based on the basic sensing function, such as mechanical, electrochemical, optical, magnetic, thermal, and so on, or they can be classified on the basis of type, application, and placement, as shown in Table 3.1.

Table 3.1 Classification of sensors

On the basis of type	Temperature sensors, blood glucose sensors, blood oxygen sensors, ECG sensors, image sensors, motion sensors, inertial sensors, pressure sensors, etc.
On the basis of application	Diagnostics, monitoring, medical therapeutics, imaging, wellness, and fitness
On the basis of placement	Strip sensors, wearable sensors, implantable sensors, invasive/non-invasive sensors, ingestible sensors

3.3 Biomedical Sensors

Biomedical sensors are sensors that detect medically relevant parameters which ranges from simple physical parameters like heart rate, galvanic skin response to muscle movements. They may be small, tiny, and often intelligent devices that are used to measure physical variables like temperature, humidity, gas, velocity, flow rate, pressure, light, electric fields, and so on. In medical diagnostics, various sensors are required for digital blood pressure meters, digital thermometers, spirometers, respiration pulse oximeters, and amongst others, location sensors based on magnetic fields.

In medicine and biotechnology, biomedical sensors are used to detect specific biological, chemical, or physical processes, which then transmit or report the monitored data. These sensors can also be components in systems that process clinical samples, such as increasingly common lab-on-a-chip devices. Miniaturized biomedical sensors are also used for measuring muscle displacement, blood pressure, core body temperature, blood flow, cerebrospinal fluid pressure, and bone growth velocity. With more and more people adopting home health care services, the demand for medical instruments that employ biomedical sensors is growing rapidly.

EMG Sensor

Known as electromyography (EMG), it is a method to evaluate motor unit action potential activity in a muscle region. As electrical signals travel through nerves to neuromuscular junctions, the change in electrical potentials (voltage) can be measured. Some current examples of the EMG sensors being used today are in virtual reality (VR) and prosthetic arms.

Galvanic Skin Response Sensor

Known as galvanic skin response (GSR), it refers to changes in sweat gland activity that are reflective of the intensity of our emotional state, otherwise known as emotional arousal. Skin conductance offers direct insights into autonomous emotional regulation as it is not under conscious control. For example, if you are scared, happy, agitated or having any emotional related response, we will experience an increase in eccrine sweat gland activity which the sensor can pick up through the electrodes and transmit to the master device.

Fig 3.1 shows a typical GSR sensor.

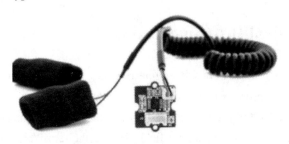

Fig 3.1　A typical GSR sensor

Heart Rate Sensor

It is also known as a heart rate monitor (see Fig 3.2). It is a personal monitoring device that allows a user to track and display his/her heart rate in real time or for studies purposes. There are two ways (electrical and optical) that this sensor monitors your heart rate.

- Electrical— consists of 2 elements which are a monitor and a receiver. When a heartbeat is detected, a radio signal or coded signal will be transmitted, which the receiver uses to display/determine the current heart rate.

- Optical— uses a light that shines through a human skin which will then measure the amount of light that reflects back. The light reflections will vary as blood pulses under the skin will go past the light which are then interpreted as heartbeats.

Fingerprint Sensor

Like optical sensors, capacitive fingerprint scanners generate an image of the ridges and valleys that make up a fingerprint. However, instead of sensing the print using light, the capacitors use electrical current. Arrays of tiny capacitor circuits collect data about a fingerprint which when connected to conductive plates on the surface of the scanner, can be used to track the details of a fingerprint. An op-amp integrator circuit is used to track changes when a finger's ridge is placed over the conductive plates which will change the charge slightly, while an air gap will leave the charge unchanged. Fig 3.3 is a picture of a fingerprint sensor.

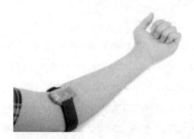 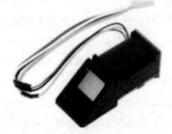

Fig 3.2　Heart rate sensor/monitor　　　　　Fig 3.3　Fingerprint sensor

3.4　Biomedical Instrumentation

Biomedical instrumentation and engineering are the application of knowledge and technologies to solve problems related to living biological systems. It involves diagnosis, treatment and prevention of disease in human. As the medical field is emerging, the area of biomedical engineering is an expanding field. We use the term "bio" to denote something related to life. When basics of physics and chemistry get applied to the living things, we name them as biophysics and biochemistry. So, when the discipline of engineering and medicine interacts, it is called biomedical engineering.

It involves measurement of biological signals like ECG, EMG, or any electrical signals generated in the human body. Biomedical instrumentation helps physicians to diagnose the problem and provide treatment. To measure biological signals and to design a medical instrument, concepts of electronics and measurement techniques are needed. Any medical instrument consists of the following functional basic parts (see Fig 3.4).

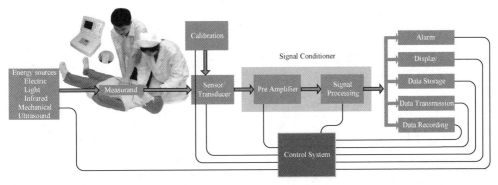

Fig 3.4   Functional basic parts of a medical instrument

Measurand. The measurand is the physical quantity, and the instrumentation systems measure it. Human body acts as the source for measurand, and it generates biosignals. A good example is a body surface or blood pressure in the heart.

Sensor/Transducer. The transducer converts one form of energy to another form, usually electrical energy. For example, the piezoelectric sensor can convert mechanical vibrations into the electrical signal.

The transducer produces a usable output depending on the measurand. The sensor is used to sense the signal from the source. It is used to interface the signal with human.

Signal conditioner. Signal conditioning circuits are used to convert the output from the transducer into an electrical value. The instrument system sends this quantity to the display or recording system. Generally, signal conditioning process includes amplification, filtering, analogue to digital (ADC) and digital to analogue (DAC) conversions. Signal conditioning improves the sensitivity of instruments.

Display. It is used to provide a visual representation of the measured parameter or quantity. Good examples include chart recorder and cathode ray oscilloscope (CRO). Sometimes alarms are used to hear the audio signals. A good example is signals generated in doppler ultrasound scanner used for fetal monitoring.

Data storage and data transmission. Data storage is used to store the data and can be used for future reference. Recently, electronic health records are utilized in hospitals. Data transmission is used in telemetric systems, where data can be transmitted from one location to another remotely.

Words and Expressions

biomedical sensor	生物医学传感器
transducer [trænz'dʒuːsə(r)]	*n.* 换能器，转换器
electrochemical [ɪˌlektrəʊ'kemɪkəl]	*adj.* 电化学的
magnetic [mæg'netɪk]	*adj.* 有磁性的，磁性的
thermal ['θɜːməl]	*adj.* 热的，热量的
motion sensor	运动传感器
inertial sensor	惯性传感器
therapeutic [ˌθerə'pjuːtɪk]	*adj.* 治疗的，医疗的，治病的
wearable sensor	可穿戴传感器
implantable sensor	可植入式传感器
ingestible sensor	可吸收式传感器
galvanic skin response	皮肤电反应
spirometer [spaɪ'rɒmitə]	*n.* 肺量计
respiration pulse oximeter	呼吸脉搏氧饱和度仪
location sensor	位置感应器，位置传感器
magnetic field	磁场
lab-on-a-chip device	芯片上实验室器械
core body temperature	体核温度，体温
cerebrospinal fluid pressure	脑脊液压力
health care	医疗保健，医疗卫生
electromyography [ɪˌlektrəʊmaɪ'ɒgrəfi]	*n.* 肌电图学，肌电图检查
neuromuscular [ˌnjʊərəʊ'mʌskjələ]	*adj.* 神经肌肉的
electrical potential	电势（位）
virtual reality (VR)	虚拟现实
eccrine ['ekrin]	*adj.* 外分泌的
heartbeat ['hɑːtbiːt]	*n.* 心跳，心搏
biomedical instrumentation	生物医学仪器
electrical signal	电信号
measurand ['meʒərənd]	*n.* 被测量
piezoelectric signal	压电信号

mechanical vibration	机械振动
signal conditioner	信号调理器，信号调节器
analogue to digital conversion (ADC)	模数转换
digital to analogue conversion (DAC)	数模转换
sensitivity [ˌsensəˈtɪvəti]	n. 灵敏度
chart recorder	图表记录仪，图表记录器
oscilloscope [əˈsɪləskəʊp]	n. 示波器
cathode ray oscilloscope (CRO)	阴极射线示波器

Key Sentences

1. In medical diagnostics, various sensors are required for digital blood pressure meters, digital thermometers, spirometers, respiration pulse oximeters, and amongst others, location sensors based on magnetic fields.

参考译文： 在医学诊断中，数字血压计、数字温度计、肺量计、呼吸脉搏氧饱和度仪及基于磁场的位置传感器等仪器中需要各种传感器。

2. Miniaturized biomedical sensors are also used for measuring muscle displacement, blood pressure, core body temperature, blood flow, cerebrospinal fluid pressure, and bone growth velocity. With more and more people adopting home health care services, the demand for medical instruments that employ biomedical sensors is growing rapidly.

参考译文： 微型生物医学传感器也用于测量肌肉位移、血压、核心体温、血流量、脑脊液压力和骨生长速度。随着越来越多的人享受到了家庭医疗服务，对使用生物医学传感器的医疗仪器的需求也在快速增长。

3. Biomedical instrumentation and engineering are the application of knowledge and technologies to solve problems related to living biological systems. It involves diagnosis, treatment and prevention of disease in human.

参考译文： 生物医学仪器和工程通常应用知识和技术来解决与生命系统有关的问题。它涉及人类疾病的诊断、治疗和预防。

Further Readings

Biomedical sensors have a vital importance in modern life. We live in an epoch of computerization for every field of life. As we all know, computers can only process the data. Data must be collected, stored if necessary, and transferred to a computer. Biomedical sensors are designed for collecting data. It might be necessary to collect data for inpatients in hospital environment, in home for homebound patients, or for outpatients. This is an equivalent of monitoring. Monitoring is a necessary activity in risky environments such as mining, diving, mountain climbing, and especially in all sorts of military and security actions. All of these broad application fields have common requirements. The biomedical sensor should be compact and should not force the wearer to leave the comfort zone. These common requirements suggest the smart (intelligent) textiles along with the notion of wearable.

The concept of a wearable device that is always attached to a person (i.e. that can constantly be carried, unlike a personal stereo), is comfortable and easy to keep and use, and is "as unobtrusive as clothing". Wearable systems are quite non-obtrusive devices that allow physicians to overcome the limitations of ambulatory technology and provide a response to the need for monitoring individuals over weeks or even months. They typically rely on wireless, miniature sensors enclosed in patches or bandages, or in items that can be worn, such as a ring or a shirt.

Wearable sensors have diagnostic, as well as monitoring applications. Their current capabilities include physiological and biochemical sensing, as well as motion sensing. It is hard to overstate the magnitude of the problems that these technologies might help solve. Physiological monitoring could help in both diagnosis and ongoing treatment of a vast number of individuals with neurological, cardiovascular and pulmonary diseases such as seizures, hypertension, dysthymia, and asthma. Home based motion sensing might assist in falls prevention and help maximize an individual's independence and community participation.

Wearable sensors are used to gather physiological and movement data thus enabling patient's status monitoring. Sensors are deployed according to the clinical application of interest. Sensors to monitor vital signs (e.g. heart rate and respiratory rate) would be deployed, for instance, when monitoring patients with congestive heart failure or patients with chronic obstructive pulmonary disease undergoing clinical intervention. Sensors for movement data capturing would be deployed, for instance, in applications such as monitoring the effectiveness of home-based rehabilitation interventions in stroke survivors or the use of mobility assistive devices in older adults. Wireless communication is relied upon to transmit patient's data to a mobile phone or an access point and relay the information to a remote center via the Internet. Emergency situations (e.g. falls) are detected via data processing implemented throughout the system and an alarm message is sent to an emergency service center to provide immediate assistance to patients. Family members and caregivers are alerted in case of an emergency but could also be notified in other situations when the patient requires assistance with, for instance, taking his/her medications. Clinical personnel can remotely monitor patient's status and be alerted in case a medical decision has to be made.

Despite the potential advantages of a remote monitoring system relying on wearable sensors like the one described above, there are significant challenges ahead before such a system can be utilized on a large scale. These challenges include technological barriers such as limitations of currently available battery technology as well as cultural barriers such as the association of a stigma with the use of medical devices for home-based clinical monitoring.

Unit 4　Fundamentals of Medical Devices

Different countries have different definitions of medical devices. General definitions of medical devices in the United States and in China will be presented here.

4.1　Definition of Medical Devices in the United States

A medical device is any device intended to be used for medical purposes. Medical devices benefit patients by helping health care diagnosis, treating patients and helping patients overcome sickness or disease, improving their quality of life. Significant potential for hazards is inherent when using a device for medical purposes and thus medical devices must be proved safe and effective with reasonable assurance before regulating governments allow marketing of the device in their country. As a general rule, as the associated risk of the device increases, the amount of testing required to establish safety and efficacy also increases. Further, as associated risk increases, the potential benefit to the patient must also increase.

Medical devices vary in both their intended use and indications for use. Examples range from simple, low-risk devices such as tongue depressors, medical thermometers, disposable gloves, and bedpans to complex, high-risk devices that are implanted and sustain life.

A medical device may be defined as any appliance, instrument, material, apparatus or other article, either used alone or in combination with other equipment/devices, including the software essential for its intended purpose by the manufacturer to be used for human beings for the following purposes of,

- diagnosis, prevention, monitoring, treatment or alleviation of disease;
- diagnosis, monitoring, treatment, alleviation of or compensation for an injury or handicap;
- investigation, replacement or modification of the anatomy or of a physiological process;
- control of conception and which does not achieve its principal intended action in or on the human body by pharmacological, immunological or metabolic means, but which may be assisted in its function by such means.

Medical devices are regulated and classified in the US as follows.

● Class Ⅰ devices present minimal potential for harm to the user and are oftensimpler in design than Class Ⅱ or Class Ⅲ devices. Devices in this category include tongue depressors, bedpans, elastic bandages, examination gloves, and hand-held surgical instruments and other similar types of common equipment.

● Class Ⅱ devices are subject to special controls in addition to the general controls of Class Ⅰ devices. Special controls may include special labeling requirements, mandatory performance standards, and post-market surveillance. Devices in this class are typically non-invasive and include X-ray machines, picture archiving and communication systems (PACS), powered wheelchairs, and infusion pumps.

● Class Ⅲ devices generally require premarket approval (PMA) or premarket notification [510(k)], a scientific review to ensure the device's safety and effectiveness, in addition to the general controls of Class Ⅰ. Examples include replacement heart valves, hip and knee joint implants, silicone gel-filled breast implants, implanted cerebellar stimulators, implantable pacemaker pulse generators and intra-bone implants.

4.2　Definition of Medical Devices in China

In China, as defined by National Medical Products Administration (NMPA), a medical device is any instrument, equipment, appliance, in vitro diagnostic reagent and calibrator, material, and other similar or relevant articles directly or indirectly contacting human body, including necessary computer software; the effectiveness are obtained mainly through physical means other than pharmacological, immunological or metabolic ways, or such ways are involved in but only play auxiliary roles, which is used to achieve the following intended objectives,

● diagnosis, preventing, monitoring, treatment or alleviation of disease;

● diagnosis, monitoring, treatment, alleviation or functional compensation for an injury or handicap conditions;

● inspection, substitution, regulation or support of physiological structure or physiological process;

● support or sustainability of life;

● control of pregnancy;

● examination of the sample coming from human body to provide information for medical or diagnostic purpose.

4.3　Types of Medical Devices

Medical devices fall into three major categories, active medical devices, nonactive medical devices and in vitro diagnostic medical devices.

Active medical device

It is defined as any device, the operation of which depends on a source of energy other than that generated by the human body for that purpose, or by gravity, and which acts by changing the density of or converting that energy. It covers all areas from dental, ophthalmic, orthopaedic and vascular, to active implantable, medicinal substances, devices utilizing animal tissue and sterile devices. Typical examples are listed as follows.

Defibrillator: to correct arrhythmias of the heart or to start up a heart that is not beating.

Electrocardiograph machine: to record the electrical activity of the heart over a period of time.

Endoscope: to look inside the gastrointestinal tract, used mainly in surgery or by surgical consultants.

Medical ultrasound: to create an image of internal body structures.

Electronic stethoscope: to hear sounds from movements within the body like heart beats, intestinal movements, breath sounds, etc.

Ventilator: to assist or carry out the mechanical act of inspiration and expiration so the non-respiring patient can do so. It is a common component of "life support".

Nonactive medical device

Examples of nonactive medical devices are orthopedic implants, surgical instruments or other sterile single-use devices, clinical thermometers, catheters, drainages, medical gloves for single use, surgical dressings and containers, etc. Typical examples are listed as follows.

Bedpan: It is a shallow vessel for patients who are unconscious or too weak to sit up or walk to the toilet to defecate.

Cannula: It is a thin tube inserted into a vein, artery or body cavity to create a permanent pathway for the purpose of repeated injections or infusion of fluids.

Catheter: It is a soft tube to drain and collect urine directly from the bladder (primary use), also to act as a makeshift oxygen tube etc.

Syringe: It is a device used for injections and aspiration of blood or fluid from the body.

Surgical scissors: used for dissecting or cutting.

Crocodile forceps: to remove foreign bodies from ear or nasal cavities.

In vitro diagnostic medical device

It is any medical device which is a reagent, reagent product, calibrator, control material, kit, instrument, apparatus, equipment, or system, whether used alone or in combination intended by the manufacturer to be used in vitro for the examination of specimens, including blood and tissue donations, derived from the human body, solely or principally for the purpose of providing information,

- concerning a physiological or pathological state, or
- concerning a congenital abnormality, or
- to determine the safety and compatibility with potential recipients, or to monitor therapeutic measures.

Typical examples are listed as follows.

Automated hematology analyzer: It can rapidly analyze whole blood specimens for the complete blood count (CBC). Results include red blood cell (RBC) count, white blood cell (WBC) count, platelet count, hemoglobin concentration, hematocrit, RBC indices, and a leukocyte differential.

Flow cytometer: It is a powerful technique for the analysis of multiple parameters of individual cells within heterogeneous populations. Flow cytometers are used in a range of applications from immunophenotyping, to ploidy analysis, to cell counting and green fluorescence protein (GFP) expression analysis. The flow cytometer performs this analysis by passing thousands of cells per second through a laser beam and capturing the light that emerges from each cell as it passes through. The data gathered can be analyzed statistically by flow cytometry software to report cellular characteristics such as size, complexity, phenotype, and health.

Urine analyzer: It is a device used in the clinical setting to perform automatic urine testing. The units can detect and quantify a number of analytes including bilirubin, protein, glucose and red blood cells. Many models contain urine strip readers, a type of reflectance photometer that can process several hundred strips per hour.

Blood gas and electrolyte analyzer: It is used in various parameters such as blood vessel hemorrhage, diabetes, drug overdose and shock for testing including hydrogen ion, electrolytes, and oxygen concentration. Blood gas and electrolyte analyzer provides accurate results for acid-base balance, blood gases, and ionized calcium.

4.4　List of Some Medical Devices

Here is the list of some medical devices classified in groups.

- **Invitro diagnostics (IVD)**

  Point-of-care testing (POCT)

  Immunochemistry

  Clinical chemistry

  Molecular

  Microbiology

  Hematology

  Hemostasis

  Immunohematology

- **Dental equipment and supplies**

  General dental

  Dental surgical

  Dental diagnostic imaging

- **Ophthalmic devices**

  Vision care

  Cataract surgery

  Diagnostic and monitoring ophthalmic

  Refractive surgery

- **Diagnostic imaging equipment**

  X-ray systems

  Ultrasound

  Computed tomography (CT) scanners

  Magnetic resonance imaging (MRI)

  Nuclear imaging

  Cardiovascular monitoring and diagnostic

- **Cardiovascular devices**

  Cardiovascular surgery

  Cardiac rhythm management (CRM)

  Interventional cardiology

  Peripheral vascular

  Defibrillator

  Electrophysiology

  Prosthetic heart valve

  Cardiac assist

- **Surgical equipment**

  Surgical sutures and staples

Handheld surgical instrument

Electrosurgical

■ **Orthopedic devices**

Joint reconstruction

Spinal surgery

Trauma fixation

Orthopedic braces and support

Orthopedic prosthetics

Orthopedic accessories

■ **Hospital supplies**

Disposable hospital supplies

Operating room equipment

Sterilization equipment and disinfectants

Mobility aids and transportation equipment

■ **Patient monitoring devices**

Vital parameter monitoring

Fetal and neonatal monitoring

Weight monitoring and body temperature monitoring

Remote patient monitoring

Patient monitoring

■ **Diabetes care devices**

Insulin pens, syringes, pumps and injectors

Blood glucose test strips

Blood glucose meters

Continuous glucose monitoring

Lancing devices and equipment

■ **Nephrology and urology devices**

Endoscopy

Dialysis

Benign prostatic hyperplasia (BPH) treatment

Urinary stone treatment

■ **Ear/nose/throat (E.N.T.) devices**

Hearing aid

Nasal splints

ENT surgical

Hearing diagnostic

Voice prosthesis
- **Anesthesia and respiratory devices**

Respiratory

Anesthesia machines

Respiratory disposables

Anesthesia disposables
- **Neurology devices**

Neurostimulation

Neurosurgery

Interventional neurology

Cerebrospinal fluid (CSF) management
- **Wound care devices**

Traditional adhesive dressings

Advanced wound care devices

Traditional gauze dressings

Negative-pressure wound therapy

Words and Expressions

tongue depressor	压舌板
medical thermometer	医用温度计
disposable gloves	一次性手套
bedpan ['bedpæn]	n. （卧床患者用的）便盆
pharmacological [ˌfɑːməkə'lɒdʒɪkəl]	adj. 药理学的
immunological [ˌɪmjunə'lɒdʒɪkəl]	adj. 免疫学的
metabolic [ˌmetə'bɒlɪk]	adj. 代谢的，新陈代谢的
elastic bandage	弹性绷带
examination gloves	检查手套
surgical instrument	手术器械
X-ray machine	X 射线机
picture archiving and communication systems (PACS)	医学影像存档与通信系统
powered wheelchair	动力式轮椅
hip and knee joint implant	髋膝关节植入物
pacemaker pulse generator	起搏器脉冲发生器
orthopedic implant	骨科植入物
clinical thermometer	临床用体温计

catheter ['kæθɪtə]	n. 导管（如导尿管）
drainage ['dreɪnɪdʒ]	n. 排水
medical gloves	医用手套
surgical dressings	外科敷料，外科用敷料，外科绷带
surgical container	外科手术容器
active medical device	有源医疗器械
ophthalmic [ɒfˈθælmɪk]	adj. 眼科的
arrhythmia [əˈrɪðmɪə]	n. 心律不齐（失常）
electrocardiograph [ɪlektrəʊˈkɑ:dɪəgrɑ:f]	n. 心电图描记器
stethoscope [ˈsteθəskəʊp]	n. 听诊器
ventilator [ˈventɪleɪtə]	n. 呼吸机，呼吸器
nonactive medical device	无源医疗器械
cannula [ˈkænjʊlə]	n.（输药等的）套管，插管
surgical scissors	手术剪刀，外科剪刀
forceps [ˈfɔ:seps]	n. 镊子
urine analyzer	尿液分析仪
analyte [ˈænəlaɪt]	n.（被）分析物，分解物
bilirubin [ˌbɪlɪˈru:bɪn]	n. 胆红素
reflectance photometer	反射光度计
hemorrhage [ˈhemərɪdʒ]	出血，（尤指大量的）失血
electrolyte [ɪˈlektrəlaɪt]	n. 电解质，电解液
acid-base balance	酸碱平衡
invitro diagnostics (IVD)	体外诊断
point-of-care testing (POCT)	即时诊断
immunochemistry [ˌɪmjunəʊˈkemɪstrɪ]	n. 免疫化学
hematology [ˌhi:məˈtɒlədʒɪ]	n. 血液学
immunohematology [ˌɪmjʊnəʊˌhi:məˈtɒlədʒɪ]	n. 免疫血液学
ophthalmic device	眼科器械
cataract surgery	白内障手术
refractive surgery	角膜屈光手术
cardiovascular surgery	心血管外科
cardiac rhythm management (CRM)	心脏节律管理
interventional cardiology	介入心脏病学
defibrillator [di:ˈfɪbrəleɪtə]	n. 除颤器
electrophysiology [ɪˌlektrəʊˌfɪzɪˈɒlədʒɪ]	n. 电生理学
prosthetic heart valve	人工心脏瓣膜

cardiac assist	心脏辅助
surgical sutures and staples	外科缝线和吻合器
handheld surgical instrument	手持式手术器械
orthopedic device	矫形器械
trauma fixation	创伤固定（器）
orthopedic braces	矫形支架
orthopedic prosthetics	矫形修复学
sterilization equipment and disinfectants	灭菌器械和消毒器械
insulin pen	胰岛素笔
syringe [sɪˈrɪndʒ]	n. 注射器
blood glucose test strip	血糖试纸
blood glucose meter	血糖计
lancing device	切割器械，采血笔
nephrology and urology devices	肾脏和泌尿系统器械
dialysis [daɪˈæləsɪs]	n. 透析
benign prostatic hyperplasia (BPH) treatment	良性前列腺增生的治疗
urinary stone treatment	尿路结石治疗
ear/nose/throat (E.N.T.) devices	耳鼻喉器械，五官科器械
nasal splint	鼻夹
anesthesia and respiratory devices	麻醉和呼吸器械
anesthesia machine	麻醉机
respiratory disposables	呼吸一次性用品
anesthesia disposables	麻醉一次性用品
neurology [njʊˈrɒlədʒi]	n. 神经学
neurostimulation	神经电刺激术
neurosurgery [ˌnjʊərəʊˈsɜːdʒəri]	n. 神经外科（学）
interventional neurology	介入神经学
cerebrospinal fluid	脑脊液
adhesive dressings	胶粘敷料
gauze dressings	纱布敷料
negative-pressure wound therapy	负压伤口治疗

Key Sentences

1. A medical device is any device intended to be used for medical purposes. Medical devices benefit patients by helping health care diagnosis, treating patients and helping

patients overcome sickness or disease, improving their quality of life.

参考译文：医疗器械是指用于医疗目的的任何器械。医疗器械通过帮助医疗健康诊断、患者治疗和帮助患者战胜疾病、提高其生活质量而使患者受益。

2. A medical device may be defined as any appliance, instrument, material, apparatus or other article, either used alone or in combination with other equipment/devices, including the software essential for its intended purpose by the manufacturer to be used for human beings.

参考译文：医疗器械可定义为以单一形式或与其他设备/装置结合使用的任何器具、器械、材料、仪器或其他物品，包括制造商为实现器械的预设用途而设计的必需软件。

3. In China, as defined by National Medical Products Administration (NMPA), a medical device is any instrument, equipment, appliance, in vitro diagnostic reagent and calibrator, material, and other similar or relevant articles directly or indirectly contacting human body, including necessary computer software; the effectiveness are obtained mainly through physical means other than pharmacological, immunological or metabolic ways, or such ways are involved in but only play auxiliary roles.

参考译文：在中国，根据国家药品监督管理局（NMPA）的定义，医疗器械是指直接或者间接用于人体的仪器、设备、器具、体外诊断试剂及校准物、材料及其他类似或者相关物品，包括所需要的计算机软件；其效用主要通过物理手段获得，而非通过药理学、免疫学或代谢的方式获得，或者虽然有这些方式参与但仅起辅助作用。

Further Readings

Top Ranked Medical Device Companies in the World

Medical device companies have experienced steady growth over the years, and it is predicted that they will continue to grow.

Medtronic is a medical device company founded in 1949. It is headquartered in the Republic of Ireland but has its executive headquarters in Minnesota as it generates the majority of its profit from the US. It started as a medical equipment repair shop. After making the first artificial battery-powered pacemaker, the repair company steadily expanded to become a huge medical device company. In 2018, Medtronic was ranked as the world's largest medical device company, operating in more than 140 countries and employing over 86,000 people.

Philips is a Dutch corporation, which has its headquarters in Amsterdam. It is one of the largest electronics company with its main focus on lighting and health care. The company started with the production of carbon-filament lamps and expanded its business to the creation of other electrical products. The company is focusing on two different areas: lighting and health care, and Philips health care is divided into two main divisions: consumer health and professional health care, with the aim of making an impact anywhere and everywhere from hospitals to home. The company is now trying to be innovative for consumers through extensive research.

Johnson & Johnson is an American multinational corporation. It was founded in 1886. And it aimed to create ready-to-use surgical dressings. With its headquarters now in New Jersey, it operates with more than 250 subsidiary companies in more than 175 different countries. It has grown to be one of the most important corporations.

Johnson & Johnson is a family of companies. It has numerous companies under its umbrella and, therefore, has been divided into three broad divisions for efficiency. The first division is consumer health care. This division mainly focuses on products that are required daily to maintain a quality of life. The second division is pharmaceuticals. This includes the production of products that are necessary for the treatment of diseases and increasing immunity. The third division is for medical devices. The company is using the majority of its resources in this division to change the treatment options and deliver help efficiently. Also, the company has been prioritizing big ideas across science to develop new devices and methods to provide care. They have been able to advance sterilization products, joint reconstruction tools, sports medications, insulin delivering devices, and many more.

Top Ranked Medical Device Companies in China

Shenzhen Mindray Bio-Medical Electronics Co., Ltd. (Mindray for short), a Sino-U.S. joint venture, located in Shenzhen, China, is engaged in the development, manufacturing, marketing and selling of electro-medical equipment in the patient monitoring, laboratory instrument and medical ultrasound fields. It is one of the worldwide leading suppliers of medical devices and solutions. Products include patient monitoring and life support systems, in vitro diagnostics and medical imaging systems, orthopaedic implants, etc.

Yuwell—Jiangsu yuyue Medical Equipment & Supply Co., Ltd. is a Chinese listed company founded in 1998. Yuwell brings professional health management concept and advanced product solution into daily life, makes a health ecosystem consisting of homecare medical, clinic medical and internet medical and builds up a professional and comprehensive medical service platform.

Yuwell's headquarters is located in Shanghai, China. It owns several R&D centers and production bases, which are spread in San Diego (US), Tuttlingen (German), Taiwan, Beijing, Shanghai, Nanjing, Suzhou and Danyang. Besides, its representative offices site over the world, reaching a complete network of R&D, production, sales and services.

Yuwell now is cooperating with Chinese famous medical agencies and core expert groups to meet and exceed health care requirements in homecare field and chronic disease management field. Several categories of Yuwell's market share have kept No.1 in three fields of respiratory system, cardiovascular system and endocrine system for many years. Undoubtedly, Yuwell is one of the top brands in Chinese homecare medical device industry.

Lepu Medical Technology (Beijing) Co., Ltd. is specialized in the design, manufacture and marketing of medical devices and equipment. Products are dedicated to cardiovascular interventions, cardiac surgery, cardiac rhythm management, anesthesia, intensive care, in vitro diagnostics and general surgery.

Shinva Medical Instrument Co., Ltd. is a China-based company principally engaged in the manufacture and distribution of medical equipment. The company's main products consist of medical sterilization equipment, cleansing and disinfection equipment, sterile supplies, sterilization and supply center project, pharmaceutical sterilization equipment, automatic conveying systems, process control management system, brachytherapy machine and others. The company distributes its products within domestic market and to overseas markets.

Di'an Diagnostics Group Co., Ltd. is a China-based company principally engaged in the provision of medical diagnosis outsourcing service. The company operates through two main segments: Service Industry segment and Business Trading segment. The Service Industry segment is primarily involved in the fields including diagnosis services, diagnostic equipment distribution, cold chain logistics and physical health examination.

Biomedical Engineers: The Hidden Heroes of the COVID-19 Crisis

Corona virus disease 2019 (COVID-19) is an infectious disease caused by the SARS-CoV-2. Most people infected with the virus will experience mild to moderate respiratory illness and recover without requiring special treatment. However, some will become seriously ill and require medical attention. Older people and those with underlying medical conditions like cardiovascular disease, diabetes, chronic respiratory disease, or cancer are more likely to develop serious illness. Anyone can get sick with COVID-19 and become seriously ill or die at any age.

Many people working in engineering have responded to the ongoing crisis by adapting their existing skills and equipment to help fight COVID-19. With the hugely increased demand for ventilators and other equipment, we have seen the important role that medical technology plays in patient care.

Biomedical engineers from a range of industry backgrounds have been putting their normal tasks to one side to build ventilators and personal protection. They are using their ingenuity to make the items that are so desperately needed. Many are using reverse engineering techniques to help them to deconstruct items and their parts to help them better understand the make-up of the equipment and the optimum methods needed to recreate them. This process would normally take many months, but the challenge now is to shorten this time frame as much as possible. Items are needed within days or weeks, so they are working to safely speed up the production and testing process, to ensure that equipment is distributed quickly, while still meeting high health and safety requirements.

One of the many processes used in manufacturing is three-dimensional (3D) printing. This is a useful tool for engineers, as it allows them to make copies of precise items several times over. In response to the COVID-19 outbreak, many small companies or individuals with access to 3D printers are doing their part to produce additional face masks and visors for health care workers, and those working in close proximity to other people.

This pandemic has helped to highlight some of the unseen professions that help to make our health service work, and show the positive impact that Biomedical Engineering in particular can have on people's lives.

Unit 5   Introduction to Hematology Analysis

Blood cells, also known as hemocytes, are cells produced mostly in the blood. Blood makes up about 8% of the human body weight . The cells and cellular components of human blood are shown in Fig 5.1.

- Blood cells make up about 45% of the blood volume, while the rest (55%) is occupied by blood plasma.

- Blood contains three different types of blood cells, namely, red blood cell (erythrocytes), white blood cell (leukocytes), and platelets.

- In turn, there are three types of white blood cells — lymphocytes, monocytes, and granulocytes — and three main types of granulocytes (neutrophils, eosinophils, and basophils).

- Blood cells are crucial for various functions of blood like transporting oxygen and other essentials, protecting against antigens, and restoring tissues in the body.

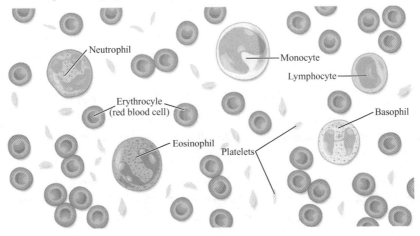

Fig 5.1   The cells and cellular components of human blood

The main functions of the blood cells include transporting gases (oxygen, carbon dioxide, nitrogen), nutrients, and hormones, helping with the maintenance of acid-base homeostasis, maintaining a constant body temperature, etc. Cells in the blood include,

- Red blood cells — round and biconcave cells without a nucleus, transporting oxygen.

- White blood cells — consist of neutrophils, eosinophils, basophils, lymphocytes, and monocytes, and they are soldiers of the immune system that fight infections and invaders.

- Platelets — derive from megakaryocytes and are responsible for homeostasis, and are something related to coagulation.

Physical properties of each cell are shown in Table 5.1.

Table 5.1　Physical properties of each cell

Type	RBC	WBC	Platelet	Hemoglobin
Number of cells per μL	Man: $(4.6\sim6.2)\times10^{12}$/L	$(4\sim10)\times10^9$/L	$(100\sim300)\times10^9$/L	$120\sim160$g/L
	Woman: $(4.2\sim5.4)\times10^{12}$/L			$110\sim150$g/L
Diameter	$6\sim9$μm	$7\sim25$μm	$2\sim3$μm	

5.1　Cellular Analysis Using the Coulter Principle

While under contract to the United States Navy in the late 1940s, Wallace H. Coulter developed a method for counting and sizing cells. The method was principally developed to count blood cells accurately and quickly. Its acceptance in the field of hematology is evident in that presently over 98% of automated cell counters incorporate the Coulter Principle. In the past fifty years, the method has also been utilized to characterize thousands of different biological and industrial materials. Bacteria, yeast cells, drugs, pigments, foods, explosives, clay, minerals, metals and many others have all been analyzed by the Coulter Principle. This method may be used to measure any particulate material that can be suspended in an electrolyte.

The Coulter Principle is based on the detection and measurement of changes in electrical resistance produced by a particle or cell suspended in a conductive liquid (diluent) passing through a small aperture. When particles or cells are suspended in a conductive liquid, they function as discrete insulators. When a dilute suspension of particles is drawn through a small cylindrical aperture, the passage of each individual cell momentarily modulates the impedance of the electrical path between two submerged electrodes located on each side of the aperture, creating an electrical pulse. Fig 5.2 illustrates the passage of a cell through an aperture.

The number of electrical pulses indicates cell count, while the amplitude of the electrical pulse produced depends on the cell's volume. The effective resistance between the electrodes is due to the resistance of the conductive liquid within the boundaries of the aperture.

Fig 5.3 shows voltage changes caused by different cells. When they pass through the aperture, (a) shows the wave before shaping, while (b) shows the wave after shaping. Note that (1) the number of pulses is the same as that of cells passing through the aperture; (2) the amplitude of the pulse is proportional to the cell's volume.

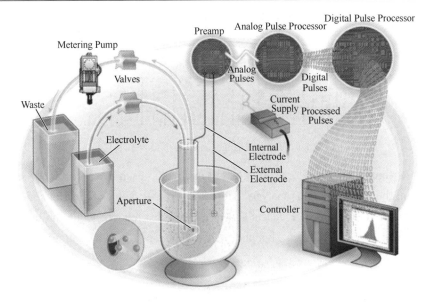

Fig5.2   The passage of a cell through an aperture

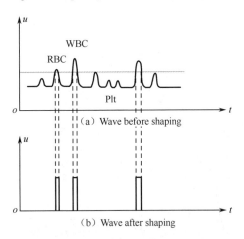

Fig 5.3   Electric pulses before and after shaping

● Set the threshold at U_1, the numbers of RBCs and WBCs will be obtained. However, the number of WBCs is so small that it can be ignored when compared to that of RBCs. Then the number of RBCs can be achieved.

● Set the threshold at U_2, the numbers of RBCs, WBCs and Platelets will be obtained. After subtraction, the number of Platelets can be obtained.

● Add hemolytic agents to dissolve the RBCs, set the threshold at U_1 again, then the number of WBCs will be obtained as Fig 5.4 shows.

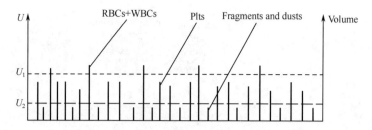

Fig 5.4　Voltage changes caused by different cells

These figures in Fig 5.5 show the histograms of each kind of blood cells after performing the cell counting analysis. Here the normal red cell distribution curve is bell-shaped, the histogram of Platelets shows skewed distribution, while the histogram of WBCs includes three parts, that is, lymphocytes, middle range cells and granulocytes.

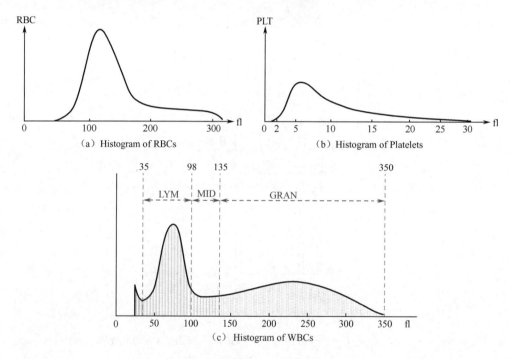

Fig 5.5　Histograms of the cells

5.2　VCS Technology

VCS (volume, conductivity, and scatter) technology measures cells nearly in their "near native state" using direct current impedance for measuring volume (V) of the cells. Conductivity (C) is measured by radiofrequency opacity to analyze the internal composition of the cells and light scatter (S) is measured by a laser beam to analyze the granularity and structure of the nucleus, as Fig 5.6 shows.

Volume. As opposed to using 0° light loss to estimate cell size, VCS utilizes the Coulter Principle of direct current (DC) impedance to physically measure the volume that the entire cell displaces in an isotonic diluent. This method accurately sizes all cell types regardless of their orientation in the light path.

Conductivity. Alternating current (AC) in the radio frequency (RF) range short-circuits the bipolar lipid layer of a cell's membrane, allowing the energy to penetrate the cell. This powerful probe is used to collect information about the internal structure of the cell, including chemical composition and nuclear volume.

Scatter. When a cell is struck by the coherent light of a laser beam, the scattered light spreads out in all directions. Using a proprietary new detector, median angle light scatter signals are collected to obtain information about cellular granularity, nuclear lobularity and cell surface structure.

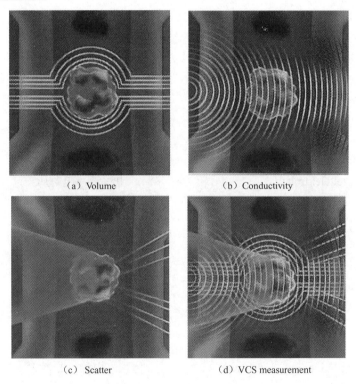

(a) Volume   (b) Conductivity

(c) Scatter   (d) VCS measurement

Fig 5.6   Volume, conductivity and scatter technology

Words and Expressions

hemocyte ['hi:məsaɪt]	n. 血细胞
erythrocyte [ɪ'rɪθrəʊsaɪt]	n. 红细胞
leukocyte ['lju:kəsaɪt]	n. 白细胞
platelet ['pleɪtlət]	n. 血小板
lymphocyte ['limfəsaɪt]	n. 淋巴细胞
monocyte ['mɒnəʊsaɪt]	n. 单核细胞
granulocyte ['grænjʊləˌsaɪt]	n. 粒细胞，有粒白细胞
neutrophil ['nju:trəfɪl]	n. 中性粒细胞，嗜中性粒细胞
eosinophil [ˌi:ə'sɪnəfɪl]	n. 嗜酸性粒细胞
basophil ['beɪsəfɪl]	n. 嗜碱性粒细胞
antigen ['æntɪdʒən]	n. 抗原（能激发人体产生抗体）
carbon dioxide	二氧化碳
nitrogen ['naɪtrədʒən]	n. 氮气
hormone ['hɔ:məʊn]	n. 激素，荷尔蒙
homeostasis [ˌhəʊmiəʊ'steɪsɪs]	n. 体内稳态，内环境稳定
biconcave [baɪ'kɒnkeɪv]	adj. 双凹面的，两面凹的
megakaryocyte [megə'kærɪəʊsaɪt]	n. 巨核细胞
coagulation [kəʊˌægjə'leɪʃn]	n. 凝固作用，凝结
hematology [ˌhi:mə'tɒlədʒɪ]	n. 血液学
pigment ['pɪgmənt]	n. 色素，颜料
electrolyte [ɪ'lektrəlaɪt]	n. 电解液，电解质
electrical resistance	电阻
diluent ['dɪljʊənt]	n. 稀释液
aperture ['æpətʃə]	n. 小孔
suspend [sə'spend]	v. 悬浮
suspension [sə'spenʃən]	n. 悬浮液
electrical pulse	电脉冲
effective resistance	有效电阻
shaping ['ʃeɪpɪŋ]	n. 整形
volume, conductivity, and scatter	体积，电导，光散射
laser beam	激光束
direct current	直流
light path	光程
radio frequency	射频

alternating current 交流

membrane ['membreɪn] *n.*（细胞）膜

lobularity *n.* 分叶状结构

Key Sentences

1. In the past fifty years, the method has also been utilized to characterize thousands of different biological and industrial materials. Bacteria, yeast cells, drugs, pigments, foods, explosives, clay, minerals, metals and many others have all been analyzed by the Coulter Principle. This method may be used to measure any particulate material that can be suspended in an electrolyte.

参考译文： 在过去的五十年中，该方法还被用于表征数千种不同的生物和工业材料。细菌、酵母细胞、药物、色素、食品、炸药、黏土、矿物、金属等都可用库尔特原理进行分析。该方法可用于测量可悬浮在电解液中的任何颗粒材料。

2. The Coulter Principle is based on the detection and measurement of changes in electrical resistance produced by a particle or cell suspended in a conductive liquid (diluent) passing through a small aperture. When particles or cells are suspended in a conductive liquid, they function as discrete insulators. When a dilute suspension of particles is drawn through a small cylindrical aperture, the passage of each individual cell momentarily modulates the impedance of the electrical path between two submerged electrodes located on each side of the aperture, creating an electrical pulse.

参考译文： 当悬浮在导电液体（稀释剂）中的颗粒或者细胞通过小孔时，将产生电阻的变化，库尔特原理就是基于对这种电阻变化的检测和测量。当颗粒或细胞悬浮在导电液体中时，它们起到分立绝缘体的作用。当颗粒的稀释悬浮液通过一个小圆柱孔时，单个细胞的通路将立即调节位于孔两侧的两个浸入式电极之间的电路阻抗，从而产生电脉冲。

3. VCS (volume, conductivity and scatter) technology measures cells nearly in their "near native state" using direct current impedance for measuring volume (V) of the cells. Conductivity (C) is measured by radiofrequency opacity to analyze the internal composition of the cells and light scatter (S) is measured by a laser beam to analyze the granularity and structure of the nucleus.

参考译文： VCS（体积、电导率和光散射）技术在细胞"接近自然状态"下使用直流阻抗测量细胞的体积（V）。电导率（C）通过射频不透明度测量，以分析细胞的内部成分。光散射（S）通过激光束测量，以分析细胞核的粒度和结构。

Further Readings

Optical Technology

The principle of optical technology is light scattering by blood cells in suspension when they pass the optical flow-cell illuminated by laser light. Using detectors that are placed under different angles relative to the incoming laser light, this technology allows measurement of different aspects of blood cells simultaneously. By correlating different optical signals generated by a single blood cell, detailed information is collected that allows for classifying the cell in a multi-dimensional space. The more information collected, the better a cell can be characterized. For example, forward scatter (very low angle) mainly depends on cell size; sideward scatter (90 degrees) predominantly reflects nuclear segmentation; and intermediate-angle scatter carries information on the presence and number of cytoplasmic granules.

Light scatter plus optical measurement of intracellular peroxidase activity through a cytochemical reaction was first used for classifying the usual WBC types. Because neutrophils and basophils cannot be separated using this approach, a second cytochemical channel was necessary for specifically measuring basophils. This optical technology with cytochemistry continues to be in use in some current hematology analyzers.

Other methods have been combined with light scatter. Initially, they used multiple channels, each with its own reagents in order to achieve the desired specificity of the WBC differential. In the latest generations of some analyzers, nuclear fluorescence is combined with light scatter and radiofrequency for constructing a five-part WBC differential.

Platelet analysis using optical technology is less prone to interference than impedance technology. Yet separating large or giant platelets from microcytic RBC or RBC fragments remains a challenge that requires additional measurements for obtaining adequate specificity. Multi-angle light scatter and fluorescent dyes have been introduced for this goal with reasonable success. Alternatively, using CD61 monoclonal antibodies conjugated with a fluorescent label provides absolute specificity to ensure reliable results at very low counts.

Principle of Light-Scatter Cell Counting

A laser beam or tungsten halogen light beam is guided at a current of blood cells that travel through a narrow channel in the light-scatter cell counters. The channel is incredibly small, causing the cells to move in one by one. When a cell is struck by the beam of light, the beam will spread at an angle. The intensity and scatter angle of the light beam differ depending on the type of cell. This is known as the cell refractive index. The refractive index is determined by the cell's form and volume while volume has the greater effect on the scatter. Sensors measure how much light is transmitted, and how much the cell absorbs from the laser.

The laser light is monochromatic, meaning it only has one wavelength, so it flies in one direction. These two features allow it to be more fine-tuned than the tungsten halogen light beam and make it more useful in diagnostic hematology for generating scatter patterns. Another drawback is that instruments with laser beams cannot be equipped with the same components as most counters. The laser counters can be calibrated only for human blood cells. Fig 5.7 is a depiction about the light scatter technology.

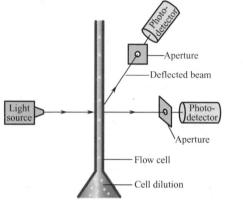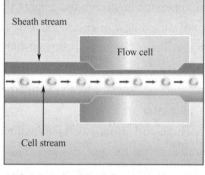

（a）Schematic illustrating light-scatter method of cell counting　　　　（b）Schematic of sheath flow, used to focus the cells hydrodynamically

Fig 5.7　Light scatter technology

Three-Part and Five-Part Hematology Analysis

A hematology analysis is usually the first test requested by a physician to evaluate a patient's health status, and automated hematology analyzers are frequently used by clinical laboratories in general health screenings.

Hematology analyzers are commonly divided into three-part and five-part systems. A three-part system differentiates white blood cells based on cell size into LYM, GRAN, which mainly constitute the NEU, but can also include EOS and BASO, and MID cells, which mainly comprise the monocytes (MONO). In addition to the CBC that can give an indication of anemia, blood clotting problem, or an ongoing infection, a three-part analyzer will also answer the question of a viral or a bacterial infection.

A five-part system, which differentiate the WBCs into all five subgroups, will provide more detailed information on conditions such as allergies and parasite infections that can be manifested as high EOS and BASO counts.

Both three-part and five-part analyzers use impedance for the RBC and PLT counts. A three-part analyzer uses the same impedance technology for the three-part WBC differential. A five-part analyzer typically uses laser-based flow cytometry for the differentiation of the WBCs, besides VCS technology. Both three-part and five-part analyzers use photometry for determination of the hemoglobin (Hb) concentration.

The Difference Between the Instrument Detection Principle

Most of the three-part instruments adopt electrical impedance detection technology, which consists of signal generator, amplifier, discriminator, threshold regulator, detection and counting system and automatic compensation device. Most of the five-part products adopt light scattering detection technology, mainly by laser source (multiple argon-ion lasers are used to provide monochromatic light), detection zones (mainly consisting of devices in the form of sheath flow to ensure that cell suspensions form a single array of cell flows in the detection flow), detectors (scattered light detector is a photodiode for collecting scattered light signals generated by laser irradiation of cells; the fluorescence detector is a photomultiplier tube for receiving fluorescent signals generated by fluorescent irradiation of cells after laser irradiation).

Three-part product divides white blood cells into lymphocytes, monocyte, and granulocyte; the five-part instrument divides white blood cells into lymphocytes, monocyte, and granulocyte (neutrophil, eosinophil, and basophil).

Unit 6　Introduction to Flow Cytometry

Flow cytometry is a technology that simultaneously measures and then analyzes multiple physical characteristics of single particles, usually cells, as they flow in a fluid stream through a beam of light. The properties measured include a particle's relative size, relative granularity or internal complexity, and relative fluorescence intensity. These characteristics are determined using an optical-to-electronic coupling system that records how the cell or particle scatters incident laser light and emits fluorescence.

6.1　Definition of Flow Cytometry

Flow cytometry is a powerful technique for the analysis of multiple parameters of individual cells within heterogeneous populations. Flow cytometers are used in a range of applications from immunophenotyping, to ploidy analysis, to cell counting and green fluorescence protein (GFP) expression analysis, as Fig 6.1 shows. The flow cytometer performs this analysis by passing thousands of cells per second through a laser beam and capturing the light that emerges from each cell as it passes through. The data gathered can be analyzed statistically by flow cytometry software to report cellular characteristics such as size,

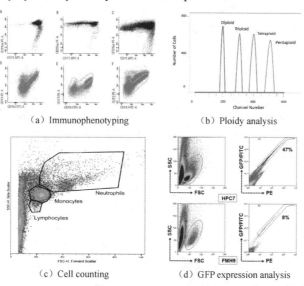

（a）Immunophenotyping　　（b）Ploidy analysis

（c）Cell counting　　（d）GFP expression analysis

Fig 6.1　Applications of flow cytometers

complexity, phenotype, and health. In this tutorial, we will look at how a flow cytometer works, how scattered light and fluorescence are detected by a flow cytometer, and how the resulting data can be analyzed.

6.2　Primary Systems of Flow Cytometer

This view shows the primary systems of the flow cytometer schematically, as shown in Fig 6.2. These are: the fluidic system, which presents samples to the interrogation point and takes away the waste; the lasers, which are the light source for scatter and fluorescence; the optic system, which gathers and directs the light; the detectors, which receive the light; and, the electronics and the peripheral computer system, which convert the signals from the detectors into digital data and perform the necessary analyses.

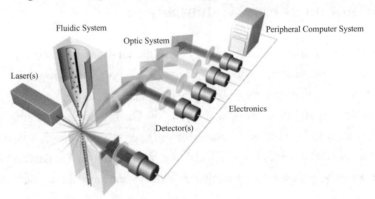

Fig 6.2　Primary systems of the flow cytometer

6.3　Interrogation Point

The interrogation point is the heart of the system. This is where the laser and the sample intersect and the optics collects the resulting scatter and fluorescence. First, let's talk about how the sample is delivered to the laser.

6.4　Hydrodynamic Focusing

Here we see how the sample is transported through the interrogation point. For accurate data collection, it is important that particles or cells are passed through the laser beam one at a time. Most flow cytometers accomplish this by injecting the sample stream containing the cells into a flowing stream of sheath fluid or saline solution. As you can see, the sample stream becomes compressed to roughly one cell in diameter. This is called hydrodynamic focusing, as shown in Fig 6.3.

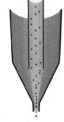

Fig 6.3　Hydrodynamic focusing

6.5　Size Comparison

In fact, flow cytometers can accommodate cells that span roughly three orders of magnitude in size. In most cases, cytometers will be detecting cells between 1 and 15 microns in diameter, although, through the use of specialized systems, it is possible to detect particles outside this range. Now let's see how laser light is used to detect individual cells in the stream.

6.6　Forward Scatter

As a cell passes through the laser, it will refract or scatter light at all angles. Forward scatter (FSC), or low-angle light scatter, is the amount of light that is scattered in the forward direction as laser light strikes the cell, as shown in Fig 6.4(a). The magnitude of forward scatter is roughly proportional to the size of the cell, and this data can be used to quantify that parameter.

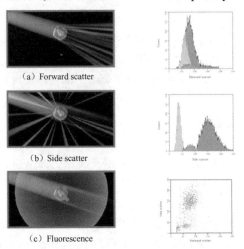

(a) Forward scatter

(b) Side scatter

(c) Fluorescence

Fig 6.4　Forward scatter, side scatter and fluorescence

6.7　Detector for Forward Scatter

But how can we record this scattered light? Light is quantified by a detector that converts intensity into voltage. In most cytometers, a blocking bar (called an obscuration bar) is placed in front of the forward scatter detector. The obscuration bar prevents any of the intense laser's light from reaching the detector. As a cell crosses the laser, light is scattered around the obscuration bar and is collected by the detector.

6.8　Forward Scatter Histogram

The scattered light received by the detector is translated into a voltage pulse. Because small cells produce a small amount of forward scatter and large cells produce a large amount of forward scatter, the magnitude of the voltage pulse recorded for each cell is proportional to the cell size. If we plot a histogram of these data, smaller cells appear toward the left and larger cells appear toward the right. A histogram of forward-scatter data is a graphical representation of the size distribution within the population, but such a graph only presents one-dimensional data.

6.9　Side Scatter Histogram

As we have already seen, a cell traveling through the laser beam will scatter light at all angles. Light scattering at larger angles, for example to the side, is caused by granularity and structural complexity inside the cell. This side-scattered light is focused through a lens system and is collected by a separate detector, usually located 90 degrees from the laser's path. The signals collected by the sidescatter (SSC) detector can be plotted on one dimensional histogram like we saw for forward scatter, as shown in Fig 6.4(b).

6.10　Scatter Plot

The one-dimensional histograms do not necessarily show the complexity of the cell populations. For example, what appears to be a single population in the forward scatter histogram is in reality multiple populations that can only be discerned by looking at the data in a second dimension. This is done through the use of two-dimensional dot or scatter plots. You can see that the peaks from the forward and side-scatter histograms correlate with the colored dots in the scatter plot.

6.11   2D Scatter Plot of Blood

Now we can view the results obtained when we create a scatter plot using forward and side scatter data from a typical peripheral blood cell run. The populations that emerge include lymphocytes which are small cells possessing low internal complexity; monocytes which are medium-sized cells with slightly more internal complexity, and neutrophils and other granulocytes which are large cells that have a lot of internal complexity. This multiparametric analysis is the real power of flow cytometry.

6.12   Energy State Diagram

Now let's take a look at another parameter that can tell us more about cell structure and function: fluorescence. As a brief review, fluorescence is a term used to describe the excitation of a fluorophore to a higher energy level followed by the return of that fluorophore to its ground state with the emission of light. The energy in the emitted light is dependent on the energy level to which the fluorophore is excited, and that light has a specific wavelength, and, consequently, a specific color.

6.13   Fluorescent Light

One of the most common ways to study cellular characteristics using flow cytometry involves the use of fluorescent molecules such as fluorophore-labeled antibodies. In these experiments, the labeled antibody is added to the cell sample. The antibody then binds to a specific molecule on the cell surface or inside the cell. Finally, when laser light of the right wavelength strikes the fluorophore, a fluorescent signal is emitted and detected by the flow cytometer.

6.14   Fluorescence Detection

How is this fluorescence information collected? The fluorescent light coming from labeled cells as they pass through the laser travels along the same path as the side scatter signal, as shown in Fig 6.4(c). As the light travels along this path, it is directed through a series of filters and mirrors, so that particular wavelength ranges are delivered to the appropriate detectors.

6.15　Fluorescence One Color Histogram

Fluorescence data is collected in generally the same way as forward and side scatter data. In a population of labeled cells, some will be brighter than others. As each cell crosses the path of the laser, a fluorescence signal is generated. The fluorescent light is then directed to the appropriate detector where it is translated into a voltage pulse proportional to the amount of fluorescence emitted. All of the voltage pulses are recorded and can be presented graphically.

6.16　Two-Color Experiment, Spectra Compatible

What if we want to do a two-color experiment? We need to look at the spectra of the two fluorophores to see if they are compatible. Alexa Fluor 488 and phycoerythrin (or R-PE) are commonly used together. For these two fluorophores, 488 nanometer light is an efficient excitation source. When excited with 488 nanometer light, you can see that the emission peaks for these two dyes are far enough apart so that discrete emission data can be collected. Compatible dyes such as these allow scientists to easily detect two colors from a single laser.

6.17　Two-Color Dot Plot

If we analyze data from the two-color experiment using a scatter plot, four distinct populations emerge. Looking at the dot plot in terms of quadrants, cells with only bright orange fluorescence appear in the upper left quadrant. Cells with only green fluorescence appear in the lower right quadrant. Cells with both bright green and bright orange fluorescence appear in the upper right quadrant and finally, cells with both low green and low orange fluorescence appear in the lower left quadrant. Multiple fluorescence parameters are necessary to dissect complex biological systems.

6.18　Filters Collect Two Colors

How does the flow cytometer collect discrete fluorescence data for the Alexa Fluor 488 and R-PE fluorophores? Filters are available that can capture the peak fluorescence from each of these molecules: a 530 nanometer bandpass filter will collect most of the Alexa Fluor 488 peak and a 585-nanometer bandpass filter will collect the bulk of the R-PE peak. Using these filters, the proportional amounts of Alexa Fluor 488 and R-PE fluorescence can be recorded for each cell. You can see that portions of each emission peak overlap one another. This is called spectral overlap.

6.19　Emission Filter Types

Let's take a moment to talk about filter nomenclature. Filters are normally defined by one of two parameters: either the center point for a bandpass filter, or the cutoff point for a long- or short-pass filter. This is a typical bandpass filter specific for R-PE. It has a center point of 585 nanometers and a width of 42 nanometers. So, this filter optimally passes light in the wavelength range of 564 to 606 nanometers, which corresponds to the emission peak of R-PE. Other filters used to resolve this peak include a 550 nanometer long-pass filter and a 610-nanometer short-pass filter.

6.20　Threshold for Forward Scatter

One final important point regarding data collection is the use of a threshold. If every single particle passing through the laser caused the instrument to collect data, the data pool would be dominated by information coming from a very large number of minute particles, like platelets and debris. To prevent this, a threshold (or discriminator or trigger) is set such that a certain forward scatter pulse size must be exceeded for the instrument to collect the data. On the histogram, the blank area represents the small cells and debris that are excluded from analysis by the threshold. This means that the majority of events that the cytometer collects are the cells of interest. It is important to realize that the small particles are still passing through the instrument; they are just being ignored.

6.21　Summary

We have come to the end of this tutorial. Our journey began with a look at the systems that make up the flow cytometer and how those systems work together to collect information on cells as they pass through a laser. We went on to examine in more detail how cytometers detect light scatter and fluorescence, and how that information can be viewed on various plots. In summary, flow cytometry is a unique tool, providing scientists with a way to gather statistical data on large numbers of cells and use that information to correlate multiple parameters within a cell population. Four- to six-color experiments are becoming easier; a few labs in the world are able to distinguish up to 18 colors simultaneously. In the next tutorial, we will talk in more detail about some of the trickier aspects of data analysis that are employed in flow cytometry, especially when two or more fluorescent colors are used.

Words and Expressions

flow cytometry	流式细胞术
fluorescence [flɔ:'resns]	n. 荧光
fluorescence intensity	荧光强度
optical-to-electronic coupling system	光电耦合系统
heterogeneous population	异质群体
immunophenotyping	免疫表型
ploidy analysis	（细胞）倍性分析
cell counting	细胞计数
green fluorescence protein (GFP)	绿色荧光蛋白
laser beam	激光束
scattered light	散射光
fluidic system	液流系统
hydrodynamic focusing	液流聚焦
sample stream	样本流
sheath fluid	鞘液
saline solution	盐水溶液
blocking bar	阻塞棒
obscuration bar	挡光棒，遮蔽条
side scatter (SSC)	侧向散射
energy state diagram	能级图
fluorophore-labeled antibody	荧光标记抗体
forward scatter (FSC)	前向散射
two-color experiment	双色实验
bandpass filter	带通滤光片
short-pass filter	短波通滤光片
long-pass filter	长波通滤光片
threshold ['θreʃhəʊld]	n. 阈值
discriminator [dɪs'krɪmɪneɪtə]	n. 甄别器
trigger ['trɪɡə]	n. 触发器
interrogation point	检测点

Key Sentences

1. Flow cytometry is a powerful technique for the analysis of multiple parameters of individual cells within heterogeneous populations. Flow cytometers are used in a range of applications from immunophenotyping, to ploidy analysis, to cell counting and green fluorescence protein (GFP) expression analysis.

参考译文：流式细胞术是一种强有力的技术，用于分析异质群体中单个细胞的多种参数。流式细胞仪在免疫表型、倍性分析、细胞计数和绿色荧光蛋白（GFP）表达分析等方面有广泛的应用。

2. The flow cytometer performs this analysis by passing thousands of cells per second through a laser beam and capturing the light that emerges from each cell as it passes through. The data gathered can be analyzed statistically by flow cytometry software to report cellular characteristics such as size, complexity, phenotype, and health.

参考译文：流式细胞仪对每秒通过数千个细胞的激光束进行分析，并捕捉每个细胞通过时发出的光。收集的数据可通过流式细胞术软件进行统计分析，以报告细胞特征，如大小、复杂性、表型和健康状况。

3. This view shows the primary systems of the flow cytometer schematically. These are: the fluidic system, which presents samples to the interrogation point and takes away the waste; the lasers, which are the light source for scatter and fluorescence; the optic system, which gathers and directs the light; the detectors, which receive the light; and, the electronics and the peripheral computer system, which convert the signals from the detectors into digital data and perform the necessary analyses.

参考译文：该视图以图表的形式显示了流式细胞仪的主要系统，具体包括液流系统，它将样本（这里是细胞）呈送到"检测点"并带走废弃物；激光器，它是散射光和荧光的光源；光学系统，用于收集和引导光线；探测器，用于接收光线；电子设备和外围计算机系统，它将探测器的信号转换为数字数据并进行必要的分析。

4. For accurate data collection, it is important that particles or cells are passed through the laser beam one at a time. Most flow cytometers accomplish this by injecting the sample stream containing the cells into a flowing stream of sheath fluid or saline solution. As you can see, the sample stream becomes compressed to roughly one cell in diameter. This is called hydrodynamic focusing.

参考译文：为了准确地收集数据，保证一次仅一个粒子或细胞通过激光束就非常重要。大多数流式细胞仪通过将含有细胞的样本流注入鞘液或盐水溶液中来实现这一点。正如你看到的那样，样本流的直径被压缩为一个细胞大小。该过程称为液流聚焦。

Further Readings

Flow Cytometry

Flow cytometry is a technology that simultaneously measures and then analyzes multiple physical characteristics of single particles, usually cells, as they flow in a fluid stream through a beam of light. The properties measured include a particle's relative size, relative granularity or internal complexity, and relative fluorescence intensity. These characteristics are determined using an optical-to-electronic coupling system that records how the cell or particle scatters incident laser light and emits fluorescence.

A flow cytometer is made up of three main systems: fluidics, optics, and electronics.

● The fluidics system transports particles in a stream to the laser beam for interrogation.

● The optics system consists of lasers to illuminate the particles in the sample stream and optical filters to direct the resulting light signals to the appropriate detectors.

● The electronics system converts the detected light signals into electronic signals that can be processed by the computer. For some instruments equipped with a sorting feature, the electronics system is also capable of initiating sorting decisions to charge and deflect particles.

In the flow cytometer, particles are carried to the laser intercept in a fluid stream. Any suspended particle or cell from 0.2~150 micrometers in size is suitable for analysis. Cells from solid tissue must be disaggregated before analysis. The portion of the fluid stream where particles are located is called the sample core. When particles pass through the laser intercept, they scatter laser light. Any fluorescent molecules present on the particle fluoresce. The scattered and fluorescent light is collected by appropriately positioned lenses. A combination of beam splitters and filters steers the scattered and fluorescent light to the appropriate detectors. The detectors produce electronic signals proportional to the optical signals striking them.

The Flow Cytometer: Fluidics

When the stained cell sample in suspension buffer run through the cytometer, it is hydrodynamically focused, using sheath fluid, through a very small nozzle. The tiny "stream" of fluid takes the cells past the laser light one cell at a time, which is called the principle of flow cytometry (see Fig 6.5). There are a number of detectors to detect the light scattered from the cells/particles as they go through the beam. There is one in front of the light beam (forward scatter or FSC) and several to the side (side scatter or SSC). Fluorescent detectors are used for the detection of fluorescence emitted from positively stained cells/particles.

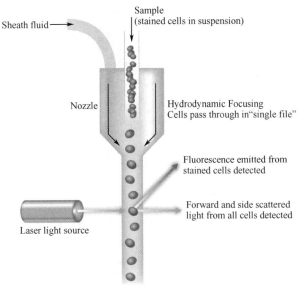

Fig 6.5   Principle of flow cytometry

Measurement of Forward and Side Scatter of Light

Particles/cells passing through the beam will scatter light, which is detected as forward scatter (FSC) and side scatter (SSC). The combination of scattered and fluorescent light is detected and analyzed. FSC correlates with the cell size and SSC depends on the density of the particle/cell (i.e. number of cytoplasmic granules, membrane size), and in this manner cell populations can often be distinguished based on differences in their size and density.

The direction of light scattered by the cell correlates to (see Fig 6.6),

- cell size (forward scatter, FSC),
- granularity (side scatter, SSC).

A useful example of this is when running blood samples on the flow cytometer.

- Larger and more granular granulocyte cells produce a large population with high SSC and FSC.

- Monocytes are large cells, but not so granular, so they produce a separate population with high FSC but lower SSC.

- Smaller lymphocytes and lymphoblasts produce a separate population with less FSC.

They are not granular cells, so also have low SSC.

Therefore, these cells can be separated into different populations based on their FSC and SSC alone.

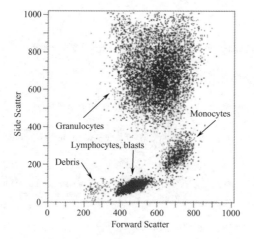

Fig 6.6   Scatter plot by FSC vs. SSC

Measurement of Scattered Light and Fluorescence

Fluorochromes used for detection/staining of target proteins will emit light when excited by a laser with the corresponding excitation wavelength. These fluorescent stained particles or cells can be detected individually and the data can be analyzed.

Forward and side scattered light and fluorescence from stained cells are split into defined wavelengths and channeled by a set of filters and mirrors within the flow cytometer. The fluorescent light is filtered, so each sensor will detect fluorescence only at a specified wavelength (see Fig 6.7). These sensors are called photomultiplier tubes (PMTs).

The PMTs convert the energy of a photon into an electronic signal — a voltage.

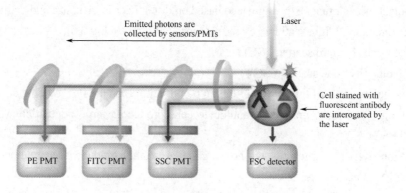

Fig 6.7   Filters and detectors

For example, the FITC channel PMT will detect light emitted from FITC at approximately 519nm wavelength. It will also detect any other fluorochromes emitting at similar wavelength.

Fig 6.8 shows an example of flow cytometer optics.

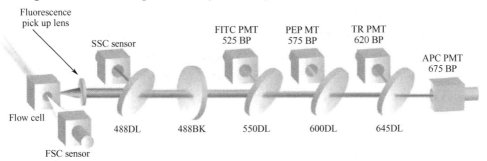

Fig 6.8   Flow cytometer optics (BP = Band Pass Filter; DL= Dichroic Long Pass Filter/Mirror; BK= Blocking Filter)

Various filters are used in the flow cytometer to direct the photons of the correct wavelength to each PMT.

(1) Band Pass (BP) filters allow transmission of photons that have wavelengths within a narrow range.

(2) Short Pass (SP) filters allow transmission of photons below a specified wavelength.

(3) Long Pass (LP) filters allow transmission of photons above a specified wavelength.

(4) Dichroic filters/mirrors (such as dichroic long pass mirrors) are positioned at a 45° angle to the light beam. In a dichroic long pass filter, photons above a specific wavelength are transmitted straight ahead, whilst photons below the specific wavelength are reflected at a 90° angle.

Measurement of a Signal

The PMT measures the pulse area of the voltage created each time a fluorescent cell provides photons.

As the fluorescing cell passes through the laser beam, it creates a peak or pulse over time in the number of photons. These are detected by the PMT and converted to voltage pulse. Each pulse for each cell is known as an event. The measured voltage pulse area will correlate directly to the intensity of fluorescence for that event.

(1) When there are no fluorescing cells passing through the optics, there are no photons emitted and no signal is detected.

(2) As the fluorescent labeled cell passes through the optics and is interrogated by the laser, the number of photons emitted increases, and so the intensity of the voltage measured increases.

(3) As each fluorescing cell completes its path through the laser beam, this leaves a pulse of voltage over time. The total pulse height and area is measured by the flow cytometer. This pulse is known as an event. Each event will have an intensity assigned to it depending on the pulse area obtained.

The pulse area is determined by adding the height values for each time slice of the pulse which is determined by the speed of the ADC, which is 10 MHz, i.e. 10 million per second or 10 per microsecond. The area is a better representation of the total amount of fluorescence.

Unit 7　Introduction to Limb Prostheses

7.1　Upper Limb Prostheses

The amputation surgery and prosthetics have historical roots back to approximately 1800 BCE. The oldest archaeologic evidence of amputation dates to 45,000 years ago. A study of a male Neanderthal skeleton found in present-day Iraq indicated that he had survived to age 40 years with an atrophic right transhumeral amputation. The topics in this chapter focus on prosthetic devices that help amputees with upper limb amputations to regain their lost dexterity and improve their ability to efficiently interact with the environment, for example, grasping an object, pushing a button, opening a door, etc. Upper limb prostheses are mainly developed to substitute a missing shoulder, elbow, wrist, and/or hand. The possible upper limb amputations are forequarter, shoulder disarticulation (at the shoulder joint), transhumeral (above elbow), elbow disarticulation (at the elbow joint), transradial (below elbow), wrist disarticulation (at the wrist joint), partial hand and finger. An image presenting all the different levels of upper limb amputations can be found in Fig 7.1.

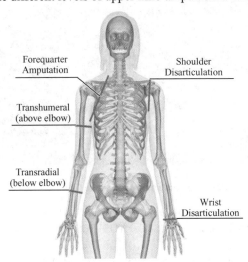

Fig 7.1　Upper limb amputation levels

7.1.1　Prosthetic Hands and Tools

Passive prostheses for the replacement of the hand include prosthetic hands and prosthetic tools. Prosthetic tools are limited to the performance of one specific activity or task that needs to be performed bimanually, while prosthetic hands can perform multiple activities and tasks. In addition, prosthetic hands appear human-like in contrast to the mechanical appearance of prosthetic tools, for example, the appearance of a passive prosthetic hook.

7.1.2　Adjustable and Static Devices

The passive prostheses can be either static or adjustable. Static prostheses cannot be moved at all. Adjustable prostheses feature an adjustable grasping or manipulation mechanism and parts of the prosthesis can be reconfigured to multiple positions or orientations. Adjustment of the prosthesis is performed by the sound hand or by pushing the prosthesis against the environment, thus by using external environmental constraints. Often little functional value for daily-life tasks is attributed to passive hand prostheses when compared to active prostheses in prosthetic research literature. Yet, user studies show that as much as one out of three amputees uses a passive prosthesis as a terminal device. An example of the passive prosthetic tools that can be used for specific activities can be found in Fig 7.2.

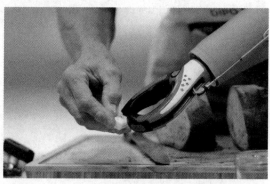

Fig 7.2　Passive prosthetic tools that can be used for specific activities

7.1.3　Body-Powered Upper Limb Prostheses

Active upper limb prosthetics can be classified into two categories, depending on the means of generating movement at the joints: body-powered and externally powered movement. They have both been in use for over 50 years and each possesses unique advantages and disadvantages. The body-powered prostheses use a body harness and a cable system to provide functional manipulation of the elbow and hand. Voluntary movement of the shoulder and/or limb stump displaces the cable and transmits the force to the terminal device. Prosthetic hand attachments, which may be claw-like devices that allow good grip strength and visual control of objects or latex-gloved devices that provide a more natural appearance at the expense of control, can be opened and closed by the cable-driven actuation mechanism. Both force and excursion are necessary to operate body-powered components. Excursion can be defined as the length that the cable needs to be pulled to operate the components, measured in inches or centimeters. Compared with externally powered prostheses, body-powered prostheses are more durable, are easier to maintain, require shorter training time and fewer adjustments, and provide more sensory feedback. However, several areas of improvements in body-powered prosthetic operation have been identified by its users, such as wrist movement and control, task completion time, coordination, and sensory feedback. The individual must use specific strategies to effectively create enough excursion in the cable to operate the terminal device or preposition the forearm in space. In most instances, glenohumeral flexion contributes the largest amount of excursion in body-powered prosthesis control. Additional excursion can be achieved through scapular and bi-scapular abduction (scapular protraction). These secondary movements allow a well-trained and skilled prosthesis wearer to increase their functional work envelope, the space in which the wearer can effectively control the terminal device. Despite some functional limitations, body-powered prostheses have provided many individuals with reliable and durable prosthetic systems. An example of body-powered upper limb prosthesis is presented in Fig 7.3.

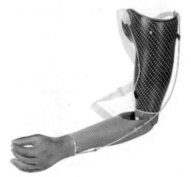

Fig 7.3   A body-powered upper limb prosthesis

7.1.4   Externally Powered Upper Limb Prostheses

The field of prosthetics has benefited from technological developments of other industries in areas of electronics, software, communication standards, batteries, actuators, manufacturing methods, material science, and mobile communication devices. Consequently, current externally powered upper limb prostheses offer increased hand dexterity, longer battery life, more intuitive control, increased function, and new methods of user interaction. The intact upper limb effortlessly performs both fine and gross motor tasks and even subtly contributes to communication. It should be remembered that the intact upper limb is marvelously capable of a minimum of 28 simultaneous degrees of freedom, with sightless proprioception (including position, heat, moisture, and pressure), with substantial strength for gross motor tasks and delicate dexterity for fine motor tasks, all with seemingly unlimited energy and unconscious control in a visually appealing, lightweight, waterproof package with self-healing properties.

For the externally powered prosthesis, the control system includes the input devices and the controller. The electronics to acquire the input signal(s) are called input devices. The controller translates the signal from the input device to the correct command then transmits the commands to the motor in the electric component. Programmable microprocessors have had a positive impact on prosthetic fitting and maximize the individual's rehabilitation potential. Before microprocessors were available, myoelectric components were designed for individuals without the benefit of real-time clinical assessment. The current technology allows the prosthetist to identify individual-specific control schemes without having to replace hardware. Benefit is derived from the ability to save, recover, and manipulate software configurations easily and quickly with immediate feedback. Prosthesis users can trial various control schemes with the ease of returning to the precise original scheme and settings quickly. An example of externally powered upper limb prosthesis is presented in Fig 7.4.

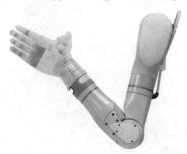

Fig 7.4　An externally powered upper limb prosthesis

7.2　Lower Limb Prostheses

The paramount aim of lower limb prostheses is to recreate the locomotion capabilities of amputees and thereby improve their ability to participate in society. Amputations of the lower extremity occur on different levels, which are displayed in Fig 7.5: hip disarticulation (at the hip joint), transfemoral (above knee), knee disarticulation (at the knee joint), transtibial (below knee), and foot amputation. With increasing level of lower limb amputation, that is, with increasing loss of parts of the biological limb, walking speed is reduced and energy expenditure is increased. Fundamentally, lower limb prosthetics are designed to increase mobility by allowing an amputee to ambulate normally. However, prosthetic limb characteristics differ from those of real limbs, for example, regarding inertia and the ability to generate work. Hence, motor functionality and economy can be significantly reduced in prosthetic users.

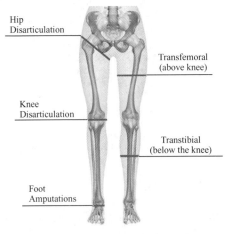

Fig 7.5   The different levels of lower limb amputations

7.2.1   Mechanically Passive Devices

Prior to 2006, all commercially available lower limb prosthetic components, including microprocessor-controlled (MPC) knees at that time, were mechanically passive (the wearer's physical effort during ambulation causes motion). Applying an analogy from upper limb prosthetics, these are body-powered designs, where all energy input comes from the user's force generation, momentum, body weight, and similar internal activation sources. For example, flexion and extension of the prosthetic knee joint occurs when the transfemoral residual limb moves the socket by means of hip joint motion. The necessary compensations to induce such motion — using the residual limb, more proximal joints, the contralateral leg, and the head/arms/trunk — have been well documented and are believed to contribute to gait inefficiency that progressively increases with more proximal levels of amputation. Lower limb prosthetic components with MPC activation have been commercially available since the release of the Intelligent Prosthesis (Blatchford & Sons) in 1990 and have been shown to offer clinical advantages compared with mechanically controlled alternatives. However, most MPC knees simply dampen motion by using software algorithms, which has a modest effect on gait efficiency. The clinical use of MPC knees became more widespread after the C-Leg (Ottobock) added effective MPC hydraulic stance stability damping in addition to MPC hydraulic swing phase flexion and extension damping see Fig 7.6. Since then, additional passive MPC prosthetic knees have become available, and the benefits of simulating eccentric muscle control during gait in this manner have been reported.

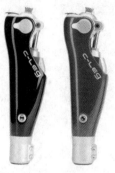

Fig 7.6   C-Leg prosthetic knee (Ottobock)

7.2.2   Active Lower Limb Devices

In 2006, Össur released the first mechanically active lower limb prosthetic component: an MPC component with a motor powerful enough to move the joint in the sagittal plane during the swing phase. The Proprio ankle/foot system (Össur) changes the plantar-dorsiflexion position of a carbon fiber foot during the swing phase to enhance gait mechanics and safety for the wearer (see Fig 7.7). For the first time, a commercially available component could simulate concentric muscle contractions to move a lower limb device. Applying an analogy from upper limb prosthetics, this was the first example of an externally powered lower limb component.

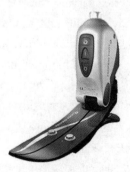

Fig 7.7   Proprio ankle/foot system (Össur)

7.2.3　Prescription of a Prosthesis

The prescription of the completed prosthesis should include socket design, skin-socket interface, suspension strategy, and additional modular components. The modular components are knee, feet, ankles, shock absorbers, torque absorbers, and dynamic pylons. The socket is the structural component of the prosthesis in which the residual limb is contained. All the forces from the ground during gait are transferred to the limb through the socket. The forces from the limb needed to control the motion of the prosthesis are transferred to the prosthesis through the socket. Much care and time should be spent on socket design and fitting, as a less than ideal fit can quickly lead to pain, injury, and lack of function. The socket design, interface, and suspension must be considered together, as their functions are often interrelated and interdependent. A soft liner, for example, can function both as an interface and as the suspension for the prosthesis. In the same way, a socket that is designed with a different interface may contraindicate certain suspension options. Forethought regarding how those three design elements intermingle will increase the probability of producing a comfortable and functional prosthesis.

Words and Expressions

amputation [ˌæmpjə'teɪʃən]	n. 截肢
prosthetics [prɒs'θetɪks]	n. 假体（人造的身体部分），义肢
archaeologic [ˌɑːkɪə'lɒdʒɪk]	adj. 考古学的，考古学上的
skeleton ['skelətən]	n. 骨骼，骨架
atrophic [æ'trɒfɪk]	adj. 萎缩的
amputee [ˌæmpjə'tiː]	n. 被截肢者
dexterity [dek'sterəti]	n. 敏捷，灵活
disarticulation [ˌdɪsɑːˌtɪkjə'leɪʃən]	n. 关节脱落，关节切断术
sound hand	健侧手
terminal device	终端设备
harness ['hɑːnəs]	n. 悬吊，背带，保护带
stump [stʌmp]	n. 残肢
latex ['leɪteks]	n.（天然）胶乳
flexion ['flekʃn]	n. 屈曲
scapular ['skæpjələ]	adj. 肩胛的
intuitive [ɪn'tjuːətɪv]	adj. 直觉的
intact upper limb	健侧上肢

proprioception [ˌprəʊprɪə'sepʃən]	n. 本体感受
lightweight ['laɪtweɪt]	adj. 轻量的，薄型的
waterproof ['wɔ:təpru:f]	adj. 不透水的，防水的，耐水的
microprocessor ['maɪkrəʊˌprəʊsesə]	n. 微处理器
locomotion [ˌləʊkə'məʊʃən]	n. 运动，探索，行进
lower extremity	下肢
transfemoral ['trænsfemərəl]	adj. 经股的
transtibial	经胫骨的
expenditure [ɪk'spendɪtʃə]	n. 支出，开支，费用
mobility [məʊ'bɪləti]	n. 移动，机动性
inertia [ɪ'nɜːʃə]	n. 惯性
momentum [məʊ'mentəm]	n. 动量
extension [ɪk'stenʃən]	n. 伸展
socket ['sɒkɪt]	n. 接受腔，穴，槽，臼
contralateral [ˌkɒntrə'lætərəl]	adj. 对侧的
dampen ['dæmpən]	vt. 减弱，抑制
plantar-dorsiflexion	跖-背屈

Key Sentences

1. Prosthetic tools are limited to the performance of one specific activity or task that needs to be performed bimanually, while prosthetic hands can perform multiple activities and tasks.

参考译文：假肢工具仅能够执行一项需要双手完成的特定活动或任务，而假肢手可以执行多种活动和任务。

2. Prosthetic hand attachments, which may be claw-like devices that allow good grip strength and visual control of objects or latex-gloved devices that provide a more natural appearance at the expense of control, can be opened and closed by the cable-driven actuation mechanism.

参考译文：假肢手可以是能提供较好握力和对物体的视觉控制的爪状装置，也可以是牺牲了一些控制功能但更美观的乳胶手套，它通过绳驱动控制机制完成打开和闭合动作。

3. It should be remembered that the intact upper limb is marvelously capable of a minimum of 28 simultaneous degrees of freedom, with sightless proprioception (including position, heat, moisture, and pressure), with substantial strength for gross motor tasks and

delicate dexterity for fine motor tasks, all with seemingly unlimited energy and unconscious control in a visually appealing, lightweight, waterproof package with self-healing properties.

参考译文：值得注意的是，健侧上肢具有至少 28 个自由度，还有肉眼不可见的本体感觉（包括感知位置、温度、湿度和压力）功能，更有控制大肌肉运动的力量和做精细运动的灵活性，在实现上述功能时，健侧上肢似乎拥有无限能量，这些功能均是无意识状态下的行为。同时，健侧上肢拥有美观性、轻便性、防水性、自愈性等诸多特性。

4. Applying an analogy from upper limb prosthetics, these are body-powered designs, where all energy input comes from the user's force generation, momentum, body weight, and similar internal activation sources.

参考译文：类比上肢假肢，就是所有的能量都来自使用者自身力量、动量、体重和类似的内部发力源的身体驱动设计。

5. The necessary compensations to induce such motion — using the residual limb, more proximal joints, the contralateral leg, and the head/arms/trunk — have been well documented and are believed to contribute to gait inefficiency that progressively increases with more proximal levels of amputation.

参考译文：产生这种运动的必要补偿（使用残肢、更多的近侧关节、对侧腿和头/臂/躯干）已被充分记录，并被视为导致步态效率低下的原因，并且截肢节段越高效率低下现象越明显。

6. The clinical use of MPC knees became more widespread after the C-Leg (Ottobock) added effective MPC hydraulic stance stability damping in addition to MPC hydraulic swing phase flexion and extension damping.

参考译文：除了微处理器控制的液压摆动相的屈伸阻尼，C-Leg（Ottobock）还增加了有效的微处理器控制的液压站立稳定阻尼，这使微处理器控制的膝关节的临床应用变得更加广泛。

Further Readings

Although the microprocessor of an externally powered upper limb prosthesis allows electric components to operate more predictably and smoothly, multiple items can interfere with their function, such as temperature extremes, electromagnetic interference, and incompatibility with the power source. Contemporary prostheses use lithium-based cells, which are smaller and lighter than nickel-cadmium batteries. The prosthetist must consider the voltage amplitude, voltage polarity, battery capacity, and electrical connections when interconnecting transducers with control systems. Additional issues that may interfere with operation of the electric components include mechanical wear and tear of the electric and mechanical components and mechanical restrictions of an aging glove. In addition, not all microprocessors are compatible with commercially available terminal devices. Therefore, the prosthetist must contact the component manufacturers to check compatibility and warranty guidelines.

All prostheses used above ankle level include a foot-and-ankle components. If the amputation is located above the knee, devices replacing the knee are added. Passive, semi-active, and active devices exist, which are categorized based on if they include mechatronic components and if they introduce forces/torques to locomotion. Passive prosthetic knees such as the Össur Mauch SNS or the Ottobock 3R80 contain mechanical linkages and hydraulics to provide damping characteristics. While these passive devices are optimized to certain gait speeds, more modern microprocessor-controlled knees, such as the Ottobock C-Leg, the Freedom Innovations Plie 3, or the Blatchford/Endolite Orion (part of the Linx system) are semi-active and can adapt their mechanical properties through actuators. For instance, the C-Leg varies joint stiffness and damping by altering the valve opening of its hydraulic component. Among commercial knee products, only the Össur Power Knee is capable of providing additional power to locomotion and it is thus categorized as an active knee prosthesis. Passive prosthetic feet are usually based on carbon springs that store energy during ground contact and release it during push-off. This basic design is also used in most semi-active and active components. Semi-active devices such as the Össur ProprioFoot, the Ottobock Triton, the Freedom Innovations Kinnex, or the Blatchford/Endolite Elan (part of the Linx system) use actuators to provide ground clearance during swing phase or align to slopes.

Part II   Special Topics on Biomedical Engineering

Unit 8   Introduction to Bluetooth Enabled FootFit Device

Chronic venous leg ulcers (CVLUs) are wounds that are thought to occur due to failure of venous return mechanisms in the lower limbs (e.g. damaged valves, past trauma from a deep vein thrombosis), which result in preventing backflow of blood and cause the pressure in veins to increase. Venous insufficiency is the most common cause of chronic leg ulceration. In the United States, it affects approximately 600,000 Americans and with the prevalence increasing with age, and 3.6% of people over 65 years of age are thought to be suffered from this.

Patients with CVLUs experience many disabling symptoms, including pain, anxiety, depression, sleep disturbance, and itching, as well as discomfort associated with lower limb swelling, tissue inflammation, and copious wound exudate. Pain in patients with CVLUs causes significant decrements in quality of life. Being absent from work, forced early retirement, loss of functional independence and unquantifiable suffering may be another additional factor that contributes to the overall burden of CVLUs. The healing process for venous leg ulcers is typically one of long duration, with median ulcer durations that range from six to eight months to those that last a year or even decades. Only an estimated 50% ~ 65% of CVLUs heal within six months of diagnosis, 20% remain unhealed after two years, and 8% remain unhealed after five years. Further, the recurrence rate is nearly 50%.

Patients with CVLUs or more severe leg ulcers are often receiving wound care, compression therapy, or various types of wound dressings for a long period of time. However, during ulcer treatment and care, the patients will encounter many problems using these traditional methods. For example, during wound care, patients experience problems, such as leakage of the wound, odor, itching, pain, the timing and the time needed or available for wound care. While compression therapy is problematic due to difficulties in putting-on and taking-off elastic stockings, or bandages being painful, too tight or coming loose, warm and itching legs on hot days, and bandages causing problems in wearing shoes.

On the one hand, since this disease occurs due to failure of venous return mechanisms in the lower limbs, it is feasible to decrease symptom associated with CVLUs and improve microcirculation and oxygen delivery by doing dedicated appropriate prescribed exercises. Such exercises may include leg elevation, pressing/pushing toes downward and upward, lifting toes upward while keeping heel firmly planted on the floor, moving forefoot like a windshield wiper, tapping forefoot up and down like keeping the beat to the music, moving forefoot like doing a figure eight, etc. Although the direct effect of such exercises on healing CVLUs is unclear, its positive effect on enhancing the microcirculation in the venules, arterioles and capillaries and hastening ulcer healing is well-documented. Most guidelines recommend three or four 30-minute sessions of each exercise per day.

On the other hand, using accelerometer is a good way to trace such physical activity or exercise because it can provide valid and reliable measurement of its duration and intensity. Accelerometer can be worn on a variety of locations on the human body, including the wrist, hip, thigh, ankle, etc. to monitor and conduct experimental studies. It has become increasingly popular due to decreased costs of the devices and good patient-provider communication network by using a handheld smartphone. Its applications include gait & posture analysis, well-being assessment, etc.

Thus, in the following section, a lower-limb physical activity training and tracking system will be presented, which is based upon 3-axis accelerometer, for the patients with CVLUs, to guide them to do all the exercises with the aim to treat underlying venous reflux, to create such an environment that allows skin to grow across an ulcer, and to accelerate ulcer healing process consequently.

8.1　Summary of Study Protocol

Study title: FootFit mHealth physical activity intervention for leg ulcer patients.

Aims: This study aims to test an mHealth intervention using wireless accelerometer technology and smartphones to promote adherence to prescribed physical activity (PA) and to encourage patient-provider communication. The PA interventions target chronically ill, very minimally ambulatory patients with venous leg ulcers (VLU).

The aims of this feasibility trial are listed as follows.

● Measure adherence (i.e. frequency and intensity of foot/toe movements, duration of each session [mins]).

- Assess patient-provider communication of FootFit and acceptability (clarity of reports, frequency and nature of patient-provider interactions, endorsement, potential for adoption).

- Conduct rigorous monitoring of recruitment, enrollment, retention, and implementation processes.

- Assess usability and refine Bluetooth enabled acceleration tracking (BEAT) technology and Smartphone applications accordingly (e.g. automated messages, patient-provider communication and confirm accelerometer sensitivity).

- Obtain estimates of variability for short-term impacts: pain, foot strength/range of motion, walking.

Major inclusion criteria: a) aged 55 years or older; b) VLU; c) ankle brachial index (ABI) 0.80 ~1.3 mmHg; d) sedentary — only able to walk no farther than 10 ft at a time; e) receives weekly wound care and able to attend all study clinic visits; f) ability to speak and write in English; g) capable of performing intervention, and h) currently not participating in a PA program.

Major Exclusion criteria: a) co-morbid conditions such as stroke; b) ulcers from other causes (arterial, diabetic, etc.); c) no 3G service in area of residence, and d) impaired cognitive status.

8.2　Overview of the System

The hardware system of the foot activity tracking device is mainly composed of a microcontroller (ATmega32L), a three-axis accelerometer (ADXL335), a low-power wireless Bluetooth (B0004) based on CC2541F256 module, a button cell (CR2032), as shown in Fig 8.1(a). These components are packaged in a small plastic box and the box is attached on a slipper worn by the subject using a double-sided Velcro, as shown in Fig 8.1(b).

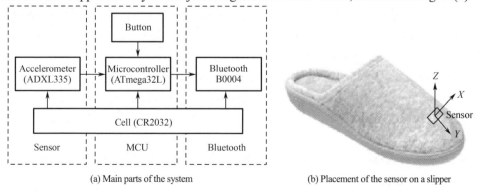

(a) Main parts of the system　　　　(b) Placement of the sensor on a slipper

Fig 8.1　The foot activity tracking device

When the patient performs a foot training exercise, the 3-axis accelerometer can detect and analyze the linear accelerations of the foot movement in three perpendicular orientations. The low consumption microcomputer coverts these analog signals into digital ones through an analog-to-digital (A/D) conversion, then sends data to a handheld device by using serial communication and wireless Bluetooth. The App, programmed and downloaded into the handheld device, such as iPhone, receives acceleration data, performs data processing, feature extraction, display, etc. Since the App is designed for the CVLUs, the App uses one click operation, that is to say only one button appears in a graphical user interface (GUI) to reduce incorrect operation and help them to finish the whole training exercises by voice tips and graphical guidance.

The rehabilitation training system for foot exercises is shown in Fig 8.2. Fig 8.2(a) shows a picture of the device containing the 3-axis accelerometer ADXL335, the microcontroller ATmega32L and the low-power Bluetooth B0004. Fig 8.2(b) shows the graphical user interface (GUI) of the App on the iPhone 5C platform. The exercise shown in this figure is the heel rotation.

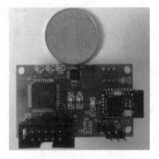
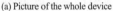
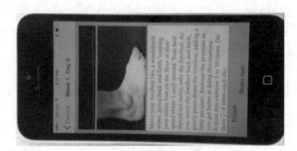

(a) Picture of the whole device   (b) The App and the GUI

Fig 8.2   Rehabilitation training system for foot exercises

Main function of the iPhone-based software includes, (1) giving prompts to enter the subject's personal information; (2) scanning and matching the possible Bluetooth device; (3) giving help to do all the prescribed exercises; (4) giving voice tips of the exercise frequency during the week, such as "this is your second exercise"; (5) extracting the features, and uploading them to the server; (6) promoting adherence of the subject to the prescribed physical activity and encouraging patient-provider communication, and reminding the subject to do the exercise every day, etc.

The subject wears a slipper with the data acquisition device on the slipper, and performs foot training exercises according to the given plan to obtain the acceleration signal. Totally, there are 3 levels of exercises, with 3 exercises on each level. These 9 exercises are dedicatedly designed to train different muscles of the lower limbs to achieve a rehabilitation purpose.

The ADXL335 is a small, thin, lower power, complete 3-axis accelerometer with signal conditional voltage outputs. The 3-axis acceleration sensor uses the gravity as the input vector to determine the orientation of the object in the space. There are angles between the accelerometer and the horizontal direction, as shown in Fig 8.3.

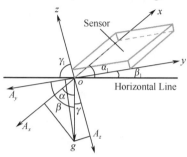

Fig 8.3   Angles between the accelerometer and the horizontal direction

Assuming that the acceleration in the x-axis is A_x, the angle from A_x to the horizontal line is α_1, and to the gravitational acceleration g is α. Similarly, the angle from A_y, which is the acceleration in the y-axis, to the horizontal line is β_1, and to the gravitational acceleration g is β; the angle from A_z, which is the acceleration in the z-axis, to the horizontal line is γ_1, and to the gravitational acceleration g is γ. With these angles, the following formulas can be derived.

$$\begin{cases} \alpha = 90° - \alpha_1 \\ \beta = 90° - \beta_1 \\ \gamma = 90° - \gamma_1 \end{cases} \tag{8.1}$$

The components of the gravity acceleration g in each orientation are:

$$\begin{cases} A_x = g\cos\alpha = g\sin\alpha_1 \\ A_y = g\cos\beta = g\sin\beta_1 \\ A_z = g\cos\gamma = g\sin\gamma_1 \end{cases} \tag{8.2}$$

According to the length of a vector, it holds that $A_x^2 + A_y^2 + A_z^2 = g^2$, the relationship between the acceleration value of the three-axis accelerometer ADXL335 and the angular acceleration value (in radian) is obtained as follows:

$$\begin{cases} \tan\alpha_1 = \dfrac{A_x}{\sqrt{A_y^2 + A_z^2}} \\[3ex] \tan\beta_1 = \dfrac{A_y}{\sqrt{A_x^2 + A_z^2}} \\[3ex] \tan\gamma_1 = \dfrac{A_z}{\sqrt{A_x^2 + A_y^2}} \end{cases} \tag{8.3}$$

Then, use the data formula: radian $= \dfrac{\theta \pi R}{180^\circ}$. This will get $\theta = \text{radian} \cdot \dfrac{180^\circ}{\pi}$. Finally, the angle values of each axis are obtained:

$$\begin{cases} \theta_x = \dfrac{180}{\pi} \cdot \arctan \dfrac{A_x}{\sqrt{A_y^2 + A_z^2}} \\[3mm] \theta_y = \dfrac{180}{\pi} \cdot \arctan \dfrac{A_y}{\sqrt{A_x^2 + A_z^2}} \\[3mm] \theta_z = \dfrac{180}{\pi} \cdot \arctan \dfrac{A_z}{\sqrt{A_x^2 + A_y^2}} \end{cases} \tag{8.4}$$

Table 8.1 shows the accelerations and the angles of the acceleration sensor when it is placed in a specific orientation. These values are used to verify whether the acceleration sensor is well soldered, and as reference for data analysis.

Table 8.1　Accelerations and the angles of the acceleration sensor

No.	Orientation of the acceleration sensor	Acceleration value	Angle value in each orientation/°
1		$A_x = -1$ $A_y = 0$ $A_z = 0$	$\theta_x = -90^\circ$ $\theta_y = 0^\circ$ $\theta_z = 0^\circ$
2		$A_x = 1$ $A_y = 0$ $A_z = 0$	$\theta_x = 90^\circ$ $\theta_y = 0^\circ$ $\theta_z = 0^\circ$
3		$A_x = 0$ $A_y = 1$ $A_z = 0$	$\theta_x = 0^\circ$ $\theta_y = 90^\circ$ $\theta_z = 0^\circ$
4		$A_x = 0$ $A_y = -1$ $A_z = 0$	$\theta_x = 0^\circ$ $\theta_y = -90^\circ$ $\theta_z = 0^\circ$
5		$A_x = 0$ $A_y = 0$ $A_z = 1$	$\theta_x = 0^\circ$ $\theta_y = 0^\circ$ $\theta_z = 90^\circ$
6		$A_x = 0$ $A_y = 0$ $A_z = -1$	$\theta_x = 0^\circ$ $\theta_y = 0^\circ$ $\theta_z = -90^\circ$

8.3   Nine Prescribed Exercises

There are nine prescribed exercises with three levels, and three exercises in each level.

- Level 1, Exercise 1: tap, wiggle or press/push toes downward into the slipper at slow speed about 1 each second. Keep your heel firmly planted on the floor. Repeat this exercise 5 to 10 times. Do them 2~4 times each day.

- Level 1, Exercise 2: lift toes upward while keeping your heel firmly planted on the floor at slow speed about 1 each second. Repeat this exercise 5 to 10 times. Do them 2~4 times each day.

- Level 1, Exercise 3: move your forefoot like a windshield wiper, going back and forth, keeping your entire foot on the floor at slow speed about 1 each second. Your heel should not move, only the forefoot. As you move the forefoot back and forth, gently press down the forefoot, adding a little pressure. Increase the pressure as you get better at doing this exercise. Repeat this exercise 5 to 10 times. Do them 2~4 times each day.

- Level 2, Exercise 1: tap your forefoot up and down, like you are keeping the beat to the music at moderate speed, about 2 each second. Repeat this exercise 10 to 20 times. Do them 4~6 times each day.

- Level 2, Exercise 2: lift your forefoot up and down, but do not tap it on the floor. You want to pull your forefoot back towards your leg at moderate speed, about 2 each second. Repeat this exercise 10 to 20 times. Do them 4~6 times each day.

- Level 2, Exercise 3: move your forefoot like a windshield wiper, going back and forth, while your forefoot is lifted off the floor at moderate speed, about 2 each second. Remember to keep your heel down on the floor. Repeat this exercise 10 to 20 times. Do them 4~6 times each day.

- Level 3, Exercise 1: push your forefoot down, like you are pressing on a gas pedal in a car. Do these exercises at fast speed about 3 each second. Do not touch the floor. Keep your knee bent and foot off the floor while you do these. Repeat this exercise 20 to 30 times. Do them 6~8 times each day.

- Level 3, Exercise 2: start with the foot lifted off the floor, and the foot at resting position (just let it hang down without any effort). Lift your forefoot up towards the ceiling, then bring it back to the resting position. This is a lifting exercise only; you do not want to push the foot down. Do these exercises at fast speed, about 3 each second. Repeat this exercise 20 to 30 times. Do them 6~8 times each day.

- Level 3, Exercise 3: move your forefoot like you are doing a figure eight, similar to the windshield wiper exercise, but gently roll the ankle around as you move your foot, going back and forth. Again, your foot is lifted off the floor. Do these exercises at fast speed about 3 per second. Repeat this exercise 20 to 30 times. Do them 6~8 times each day.

Unlike those accelerometers worn on the wrist, hip, thigh, or ankle, the accelerometer here is placed above the big toe on the slipper using Velcro to monitor and conduct all experimental exercises. It could give duration and intensity of each exercise. By using the system, it could help the older patients to adhere to all the exercises by establishing a good patient-provider communication via an App. It could be implemented as a useful method to accelerate ulcer healing process, addition to traditional wound care, compression therapy, and wound dressing.

Words and Expressions

chronic venous leg ulcer	慢性下肢静脉性溃疡
venous return mechanism	静脉回流机制
lower limb	下肢
vein thrombosis	静脉血栓
wound care	伤口护理
compression therapy	加压疗法
wound dressing	伤口敷料
elastic stockings	弹力袜
microcirculation	*n.* 微循环
bandage ['bændɪdʒ]	*n.* 绷带
accelerometer [əkˌseləˈrɒmɪtə]	*n.* 加速度计
handheld smartphone	手持智能手机
gait & posture analysis	步态与姿势分析
well-being assessment	健康评估
ankle brachial index	踝臂指数

Key Sentences

1. Chronic venous leg ulcers (CVLUs) are wounds that are thought to occur due to failure of venous return mechanisms in the lower limbs (e.g. damaged valves, past trauma from a deep vein thrombosis), which result in preventing backflow of blood and cause the pressure in veins to increase.

参考译文：慢性下肢静脉溃疡（CVLUs）是指由于下肢静脉回流机制失效（如瓣

膜受损、深静脉血栓形成造成的创伤）而导致的伤口，该伤口阻止了血液回流并导致静脉内压力升高。

2. Patients with CVLUs experience many disabling symptoms, including pain, anxiety, depression, sleep disturbance, and itching, as well as discomfort associated with lower limb swelling, tissue inflammation, and copious wound exudate.

参考译文： 慢性下肢静脉溃疡患者经历许多致残症状，包括疼痛、焦虑、抑郁、睡眠障碍和瘙痒，以及与下肢肿胀、组织炎症和大量伤口渗出物相关的不适。

3. This study aims to test an mHealth intervention using wireless accelerometer technology and smartphones to promote adherence to prescribed physical activity (PA) and to encourage patient-provider communication. The PA interventions target chronically ill, very minimally ambulatory patients with venous leg ulcers (VLU).

参考译文： 本研究的目的是测试使用无线加速度计技术和智能手机的移动健康干预措施，以增加对规定体力活动（PA）的坚持程度，加强患者与医疗机构沟通。这种体力活动（PA）旨在对活动能力极低、患有下肢静脉性溃疡（VLU）的慢性病患者进行干预。

Further Readings

Chronic Venous Disease

What is chronic venous disease? That is a question that many people ask. The patients may have had problems like swelling for many years and they notice their skin is starting to change colors, such as turning brown or getting hard or red and flaky. Chronic venous disease, which is a disorder, is a problem with the veins of your lower legs and connecting veins which connect the deep veins and superficial veins. And veins, as you know, bring blood up out of the legs to circulate it back through the body. Veins can be damaged from traumas. For example, if you've ever got a kick in the leg or you've had some kind of break fracture of your bone, and when the damage disrupts the blood vessels, those veins may not work properly. If you have problems with the large muscle in your leg, for example, when the calf muscle doesn't work well, then the veins cannot help the circulation out of your legs. Those calf muscles have to press and squeeze on the veins to get the blood moving out of your legs. So, if your calf is weak, or you have very stiff ankles from arthritis and you can't move your foot which then causes the calf not working properly, then the veins are not squeezed and pushed to transport the blood up out of the legs. Now I know this sounds very complicated, but I want you to understand that part of the disease that you have is related to other conditions that you have. And if your calf muscle in the back of your leg doesn't work well or if your ankle doesn't flex, maybe it is because you do not have good flexibility caused by arthritis or maybe you've had an injury, or else maybe your feet swell a lot that causes problems with circulating the blood in your veins. I also describe that injury could have damaged the veins in your leg, and therefore, they don't work well. These are some of the common reasons why people have problems with the vein circulation, again, which we call chronic venous disease or chronic venous insufficiency.

What Is Compression Therapy?

Compression therapy is the process by which pressure is applied evenly over a sore or painful area, squeezing to support the veins. This type of treatment usually comes in the form of tight stockings or socks that are worn during the day and removed at night.

Though it may seem counterintuitive, the pressure applied during this period through compression doesn't slow blood flow — it increases it. The improved circulation can help to promote healing and the pressure prevents blood from pooling in the veins. This process can also reduce swelling in the affected body part.

Compression therapy is the mainstay of treatment of venous leg ulcers (VLU). Good wound care and compression therapy will heal majority of small venous ulcers of short duration. Goals of compression therapy are ulcer healing, reduction of pain and edema, and prevention of recurrence. Compression is used for VLU and narrows veins and restores valve competence and reduces ambulatory venous pressure, thus reducing venous reflux.

Compression therapy, together with modern moist wound treatment, is the basis for a successful conservative treatment of patients with chronic leg ulcers. In clinical practice, it is often the patients themselves who apply compression therapies. Many of the mostly elderly patients, however, are not able to reach their legs and feet due to movement restrictions, such as arthritis, arthrosis and even obesity. An adequate compression therapy also requires extensive experience and regular training. In practice, only the minority of patients can perform bandaging well and therefore this should not be recommended. Self-management with do-it-yourself medical devices will become more and more important in the future. In addition to the psychological factors, cost aspects and demographic change, an expected lack of qualified nursing staff due to the number of elderly patients who are potentially in need of care means that self-management is becoming increasingly more important.

Bluetooth enabled FootFit device is such kind of medical device, that may be good for chronic venous leg ulcers. The physical activities designed target chronically ill, very minimally ambulatory patients with venous leg ulcers.

Leg Elevation

It is very important to keep your legs elevated as much as possible, if you are standing, or working, and you find that your legs begin to ache and you have swelling. It is very important for you to spend some time at least thirty minutes every day elevating your legs. The best way to do this is to lay down on the bed or couch. If you have a bunch of pillows, just prop up your legs as high as you can get them. Again, thirty minutes is well we recommend, and the reason why it is so important to do this is to decrease the swelling in the legs, and it helps with the circulation of getting the veins to return the blood back into the body so that it can be re-circulated. You will find that this helps with swelling and some of the itchiness and heaviness you might experience. We also know that it helps with healing venous ulcers.

Unit 9   Computer-Assisted Orthopaedic Surgery

9.1   Basics of Computer-Assisted Orthopaedic Surgery

Computer-assisted orthopaedic surgery (CAOS) aims at improving the perception that a surgeon has of the surgical field and the operative manipulation that he/she carries out. Conventional surgical handwork requires competences such as dexterity or fine motor skills, which are complemented by visual and tactile feedback. Current CAOS systems offer enhanced visualization by displaying a virtual model of the operated anatomy together with relevant information about the position of a surgical instrument or implant on a computer monitor thus improving the surgeon's visual feedback by complementing the direct visual impression of the operation site. They present greater details, three-dimensional views or sights of internal structures, which are invisible to the naked eye. The anticipated effect on surgical performance is manifold: the increased visual perception of the operator leads to an increased precision with which surgical tasks can be carried out. Bony manipulation such as drilling, chiseling, or sawing can be performed more accurately and implants can be placed more exactly. This chapter will present the basic elements that are common to all navigation systems and will describe optional features that have been implemented in the products of some manufacturers or the prototypes of some researchers.

Building Blocks of a CAOS System

The core of each CAOS system presents virtual representations of the operated anatomy and the performed surgical action and ensures, by linking this virtual model to the operated patient, that the replayed scene matches with what is performed at the surgical situs. The following subsections will explain the building blocks that make such systems reality and will present a review of available technologies.

Appropriate Patient Anatomy Representation

Operating with the support of a surgical navigation system requires an image of the treated anatomy to be used as virtual object. A large variety of image modalities can potentially be employed for this purpose, but not all of them are ideal for use in CAOS. Using established methods of medical imaging is surely most obvious and, consequently, the

CAOS systems of the first generation used preoperative computed tomography (CT) scans to represent the bone structures that were involved in the respective surgery. CTs are an almost ideal preoperative image modality for the needs of CAOS: they present the outer shape and inner structures of bony anatomy with high resolution and good contrast and without any geometrical distortions. The same is true for preoperative, conventional X-rays. Their geometrical imprecision and the fact that they capture only a two-dimensional (2D) projection of a three-dimensional (3D) scene have made developers refrain from building navigation systems based on X-rays.

In any case when a preoperative image serves as a virtual object, a so-called registration or matching procedure is required to align the operated anatomy with its preoperative image, assuming that the represented topology of the bone has not changed between image acquisition and surgical intervention. Numerous registration approaches have been described. Each of them requires certain features to be interactively or semi-automatically identified in both the patient's anatomy and the image. Based on the inherent knowledge of correspondence between these feature sets, the spatial relation between virtual object and operated anatomy is extrapolated. While feature extraction from the image dataset is performed either "manually" using the computer mouse or with the help of image processing algorithms, intraoperative digitization of the corresponding features is done by the surgeon using a digitizing stylus, laser scanners, ultrasound probes, fluoroscopic imaging or similar devices. Since the perfect alignment of image and reality is crucial for the accuracy of the subsequently available navigation feedback, this usually interactive step requires careful execution and, as an element of safety, subsequent verification of the achieved result.

As an alternative that goes entirely without "classical" radiological images, so-called "image-free" systems construct virtual models of the operated anatomy exclusively based on interactively acquired position data. Such data is either recorded by digitization methods as described above for the registration of preoperative images or is derived from the kinematic analysis of joint motion, which lets the CAOS system determine, e.g. the rotation center or axis of a joint. Resulting models are rather abstract since they are constructed from very sparse data only. To improve the realism with which the surgical field is represented on the screen, statistical shape atlases can be combined with the recorded data.

Passive Navigation Systems

Passive navigation systems utilizing a device called tracker to determine the spatial 3D positions and orientations of objects in real time. Different physical modalities have been investigated and used to remotely sense the spatial location of objects. Nowadays optical tracking is by far the most commonly used tracking modality. It utilizes infrared light that is either actively emitted or passively reflected from the tracked objects. The basic principles of navigation are outlined in the following using an optical tracking system.

To track objects such as surgical instruments or the patient anatomy, light emitting or reflecting markers are rigidly attached to the tracked objects. A system consisting of an object to be tracked and markers rigidly attached to it is called "rigid body". The optical trackers, also known as cameras, detect the reflected or emitted light signals and reconstruct the corresponding markers' 3D positions in the camera's coordinate system. From mathematics, it is known that the positions of three non-collinear marker positions are required to uniquely define the 3D position and orientation of an object in space. Therefore, the markers are usually grouped in rigid constellations of three or more, forming their own local coordinate system. By increasing the number of markers together with an optimized spatial arrangement, the visibility of a tracked object can be improved. Additionally, it has been shown that increasing the number of markers on a rigid body up to six improves the navigation accuracy significantly. With increasing number of markers, the accuracy gradually converges against a maximum.

By means of calibration or registration, the real object geometry will be defined in the local rigid body coordinate system. Knowing the individual marker positions of a rigid body and the orientation of the real object within the local rigid body coordinate system, the absolute position and orientation of the real object in the camera coordinate system can be computed. If more than one object is tracked simultaneously by the camera, the relative positions of all tracked objects can be determined as well. For tracked patient anatomies, similar mechanisms are used. By the help of mechanical supports (e.g. dynamic reference body, DRB), a marker constellation will be rigidly attached to the anatomy during the surgical intervention. As long as the marker arrangement stays rigid in relation to the anatomy, the rigid body concept is not violated and the relative position between patient anatomies and/or surgical tools can be computed. Fig 9.1 illustrates this tracking concept by showing the individual transformations between the camera coordinate system (C-cos), the tool coordinate system (T-cos) and a DRB attached to a patient anatomy forming a rigid body and defining a local coordinate system (A-cos).

Fig 9.1 shows the optical navigation system, depicting the relationships between the camera coordinate system (C-cos), a tool coordinate system (T-cos), and an anatomy coordinate system (A-cos). After the dynamic reference base is attached, the DRB and the patient anatomy are considered to be a single rigid body.

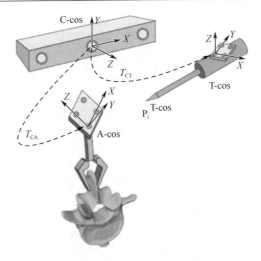

Fig 9.1   Optical navigation system

Visualization for CAOS Systems

After the introduction of patient anatomy representations with their implicit or explicit registrations and real-time tracking methods for objects together with the rigid body concept, nearly all building blocks necessary for a computer-assisted surgery system have been explained. In a last step, the individual parts are put together with visualization techniques to form a complete CAOS system. This section introduces common visualization concepts used in CAOS systems.

In general, the visualization type is driven by the clinical application. The classical visualization in CAOS systems is based on arbitrarily cut slices through volumetric data sets such as CT data. During a surgical planning step, the slices' positions and orientations can be changed by user interaction in order to plan, for example, implant positions or trajectories for fixation screws. During a subsequent navigation step, the slice positions within the slice stack are continuously updated, for example, by the tip of a tracked surgical tool using the real-time position updates from the tracking system. The surgical tools or additional information from a previous planning step like screw positions are then displayed as overlays on top of the rendered slices. Fig 9.2 shows typical CT data-based planning and navigation applications. CAOS systems utilize volume rendering techniques just to provide an anatomy overview based on down-sampled volumetric data sets. The lower right view in Fig 9.2 demonstrates a view of a volume rendered skull used in a planning application.

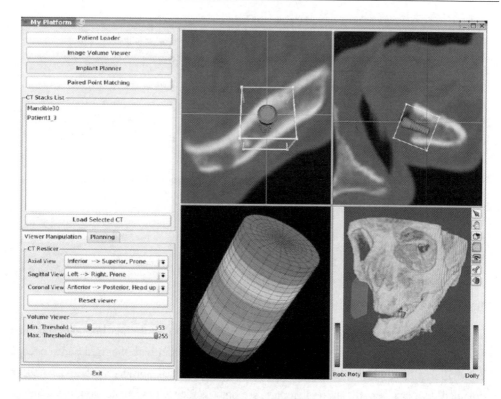

Fig 9.2 Typical CT data-based planning application showing an implant positioned as overlay on top of arbitrary slices across a CT data set

9.2 CT-Based Navigation Systems

This overview identifies the most important technical components of CT-based CAS systems, using the example of the HipNav system. HipNav (CASurgica, Inc.) is the surgical navigation system developed initially to address the problem of cup alignment in total hip replacement.

Image Segmentation, Preoperative Planning and Simulation

Because of its relatively high accuracy and the bone imaging characteristics, CT scans are very suitable for surgical navigation, especially in orthopaedics. The bones can be easily distinguished from any other tissue, and can be easily segmented out. The bones are also the least deformable parts of the body, and therefore the most stable references for navigation, making it possible for different phases of surgical planning and execution to be performed well after the patient imaging.

Preoperative planning is typically done in three orthogonal cross-sectional views made through the CT scan volume. The target bone can also be visualized as a three-dimensional object and rendered in the perspective view from an arbitrary viewpoint, which can be useful in some planning and navigation tasks. In order to create this kind of renderings, the organs and tissues of interest need to be segmented out from the rest of the image, and their boundaries have to be determined. Surface models are then built, which describe the surface of the bone of interest as a contiguous set of triangles fully encompassing the bone's volume.

Early applications of image-guided surgery where the goal is to accurately and precisely reach the target and to choose the access trajectory so that the damage to the collateral tissue is minimized (such as tumor removal, fracture stabilization and biopsy tasks) were fairly simple from the planning point (see Fig 9.3).

Planning is performed with respect to the anatomic coordinate systems derived from the anatomic landmarks. In the pelvis, the anterior pelvic plane is defined with the most anterior points — anterior iliac spines and the mid-pubis symphysis point. In the femur, the reference system is defined with the center of the femoral head and the plane defined by the lesser trochanter and the posterior condyles. After the landmarks are automatically detected in the planner, the alignment of implant components can be uniquely defined. The surgeon selects the implant components from the database and places them in a desired position and orientation, using both cross-sectional CT views and 3D surface models. In the final stage, the virtual replacement joint is assembled and tested for the range of motion simulation. The range of motion analysis is performed for any desired leg motion path, to test the impingement limits of that motion. Both prosthetic and bone impingent limits are detected. The effects of the change of any relevant parameter (orientation, size, position, pelvic flexion) on ROM and on component offset and leg length can be examined in real time, helping surgeon in optimizing the plan. The implants orientation can be modified, or alternative components can be selected, so that the safe range of motion is maximized, and the leg length change is properly considered. Once the surgical plan is developed, it becomes a blueprint for surgical intervention.

Intraoperative Steps

Tracking

The key component of surgical navigation is the ability to determine accurately and precisely at every step where the target bones and surgical tools are in space and how their position corresponds to the preoperative image that was used for planning. This is typically achieved by using tracking systems and by rigidly attaching tracking markers to bones of interest and to the surgical tools, and by tracking those markers using localizing devices (see Fig 9.4).

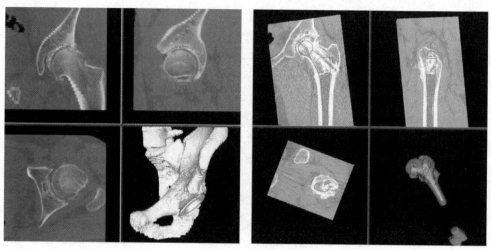

Fig 9.3   Applications of image-guided surgery: planning of the cup implant; planning of the femoral implant

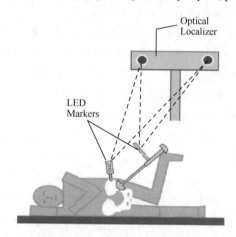

Fig 9.4   Tracking system: optical localizer tracks the positions of markers attached to a bone and a surgical tool

The most commonly used tracking systems are the optical and electromagnetic ones. The optical localizers consist of two (Polaris, NDI, Ontario, Canada) or three (OptoTrak, NDI, Ontario) CCD cameras placed in the rigid enclosure that detect the position of either infrared light emitting diode markers (active) or reflective spherical markers (passive) in space. Typically, four to six markers are placed on one rigid object, called dynamic reference body (DRB), allowing calculation of the 6 degree of freedom position of that object in space. If a DRB is then attached rigidly to another object such as medical instrument or bone, one can inherently track the position of those objects in space, as well. The orientation of tools relative to the bone of interest can then be calculated and compared to the planned one.

Registration

In order to implement the surgical plan, the position of the patient's bone in the operating room has to be correlated with the position of the same bode in the plan image. This involves finding the geometric transformation that would map the patient's intra-operative position to coincide with the position in the plan space. The calculation of this position is called registration. The simplest registration is the fiducial registration. It involves the insertion of fiducials (implanted physical markers) into the bone before a 3D image (CT scan) is obtained, and keeping them inserted throughout the surgical procedure. The fiducial markers are designed to be clearly and easily identified both in the image space and in the tracker space during the surgery. Three such markers placed in predetermined anatomical areas are sufficient for registration. Although this type of registration is conceptually and computationally simple, it requires that additional screws are placed in bone for their attachment, typically several days before surgery, causing inconvenience and increasing the risk of infection, and whenever possible this method is being replaced with alternative methods.

Shape based registration is one of the alternatives to fiducial registration, in which the shape of the part of the bone surface is measured intraoperatively and matched to the surface model developed from the CT scan. Intraoperative shape measurement of the bone surface can be done by a tracked point probe, an ultrasound probe or a laser range scanner.

Navigation

Once the tracking is established and the registration is performed, the surgeon can learn at any time what is the position of tracked surgical tools relative to the target bones, and how does it compare to the planned one. The computer interfaces then enable the surgeon to interactively reposition the tools in order to match the planned positions and trajectories and in effect assist them in navigating the patient's anatomy. Typical interfaces show the tools' current position in the cross sections through the patient's image, or as a three-dimensional view from the chosen point of view. Simple interfaces similar to those used by airplane pilots guide the surgeon to desired tool alignment.

Words and Expressions

orthopaedic [ˌɔːθəˈpiːdɪk]   *adj.* 骨科的
perception [pəˈsepʃən]   *n.* 感知

operative manipulation	手术操作
visual and tactile feedback	视觉及触觉反馈
anatomy [ə'nætəmi]	*n.* 解剖
surgical instrument	手术器械
surgical navigation system	手术导航系统
image modality	图像模式，图像形态
preoperative [pri'ɒpərətɪv]	*adj.* 术前的
registration [ˌredʒə'streɪʃən]	*n.* 配准
algorithm ['ælgərɪðəm]	*n.* 算法
intraoperative [ˌɪntrə'ɒpərətɪv]	*adj.* 术中的
joint motion	关节活动
optical tracking	光学跟踪
position and orientation	位置和定向
total hip replacement	全髋关节置换
tumor removal	肿瘤去（切）除
fracture stabilization	骨折固定
biopsy ['baɪɒpsi]	*n.* 活体标本检查
infection [ɪn'fekʃən]	*n.* 感染

Key Sentences

1. Computer-assisted orthopaedic surgery (CAOS) aims at improving the perception that a surgeon has of the surgical field and the operative manipulation that he/she carries out.

参考译文：计算机辅助骨科手术致力于增强医生对手术区域的感知程度并促进手术操作水平的提升。

2. A large variety of image modalities can potentially be employed for this purpose, but not all of them are ideal for use in CAOS.

参考译文：有多种模式的图像可用于实现该目标，但并非每种模式都是计算机辅助骨科手术的最佳选择。

3. In any case when a preoperative image serves as a virtual object, a so-called registration or matching procedure is required to align the operated anatomy with its preoperative image, assuming that the represented topology of the bone has not changed between image acquisition and surgical intervention.

参考译文：无论在任何情况下将术前图像作为虚拟模型，配准或对齐的过程都是必需的，该过程将待手术解剖部位与其对应的术前图像进行对齐，以确保骨骼的拓扑结构在图像获取和手术干预期间不发生改变。

Further Readings

C-Arm-Based Navigation

Navigation Without Manual Registration/Direct Navigation

Navigation on one or more C-arm 2D projection images acquired intraoperatively or on intraoperatively acquired 3D image data sets from the ARCADIS Orbic 3D C-arm. This simplifies the workflow compared to navigation with manual registration, and the surgical intervention can be carried out as a less invasive procedure.

Step 1: *Tracking*. The surgical instruments are fitted with active or passive markers and are tracked by a camera.

Step 2: *Referencing*. A reference marker is attached to the patient in the OR. This is to allow automatic detection of and compensation for relative movements of the patient and the camera.

Step 3: *Image acquisition and transfer*. Images are taken using the C-arm and loaded into the navigation computer. For this purpose, the C-arm is equipped with active or passive markers and is tracked by the camera during image acquisition. This means that there is no need for manual registration.

Step 4: *Navigation*. The surgical instrument is displayed as a virtual instrument (as an animated object) in the medical images in real time.

Direct Navigation in Two-Dimensional Projection Images

A common feature of both techniques of direct navigation, i.e. 2D and 3D navigation, is that the navigation system's camera tracks not only the surgical instrument but also the C-arm representing the imaging system. In direct 2D-navigation a device with the following functions is attached to the image intensifier of the C-arm (see Fig 9.5),

- Making the C-arm visible to the navigation system. The attachment is fitted with either active or passive markers. This enables the navigation system's camera to detect the position of the C-arm from which an X-ray image is being taken. Through the use of calibration, the location and the relative position of the projection image are therefore known.

- Compensating for image distortion in the image intensifier. The electron optics and the earth's magnetic field causes images to be distorted in 2D projections. The magnitude of these distortions is determined using a metal marker plate in front of the input window of the image intensifier. Compensation is performed by software.

● Online or offline calibration of the mechanical twisting of the C-arm. Calibration is necessary because the C-arm is subject to mechanical twisting in different ways depending on its position. This intrinsic movement of the C-arm is measured with the help of a two-plate attachment to the image intensifier either intraoperatively during image acquisition (online calibration) or once only during installation of the navigation system on the C-arm (offline calibration) and is taken into account in the software. With the given reproducibility of the twisting, the advantage of offline calibration is that the distance between the patient and the image intensifier is hardly reduced during surgery. In this case, only the metal marker plate that compensates for the image distortion in the image intensifier is used intraoperatively.

Direct 2D navigation can be carried out with both isocentric and non-isocentric C-arms.

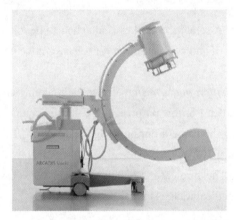

Fig 9.5   Conventional C-arm with navigation attachment for direct 2D navigation

Direct Navigation in Three-Dimensional Image Data

3D Imaging with an Isocentric Mobile C-Arm

ARCADIS Orbic 3D makes 3D imaging possible as a result of its isocentric design and 190° orbital motion supported by its hidden cable routing. In contrast with non-isocentric C-arms, the central beam always crosses the center of rotation of the C-arm during the orbital movement, irrespective of the orbital angle (see Fig 9.6). This means that the region of interest (ROI) always remains in the cone angle, regardless of the current projection angle, allowing a 3D image data set to be generated around the isocenter.

Automatic Registration

During installation of the navigation system, the correlation between the 3D reconstruction volume and a special reference point on the C-arm is determined in an offline calibration procedure. The reference point can be located by the navigation system's camera because there is a fixed correlation between this point and the active or passive markers on a marker ring attached to the C-arm. During 3D image acquisition, the navigation system's camera detects the position of the reference point with the aid of the marker ring. Because of the measurements taken during offline calibration, the navigation system's computer immediately knows the position and orientation of the 3D data cube in the OR. The position of the surgical instrument — which is tracked by the same camera during the surgical procedure — can therefore be displayed in real-time as a virtual object in the 3D image data set without manual registration. Direct 3D navigation with ARCADIS Orbic 3D is shown in Fig 9.7.

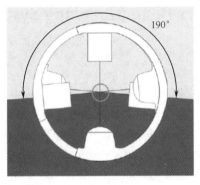

Fig 9.6   The isocentric mobile C-arm ARCADIS Orbic 3D can be rotated by 190°

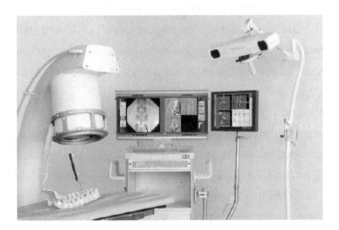

Fig 9.7   Direct 3D navigation with ARCADIS Orbic 3D

Unit 10　Minimally Invasive Surgery and Navigation: Total Knee Arthroplasty

10.1　The Surgetics Bone-Morphing System

Introduction

Total knee replacement is a challenge that aims at achieving a pain free, stable, and mobile joint. Both mobility and stability are essential for long term survivorship of the implants and this can only be achieved if the implants are properly aligned with the mechanical axis of the lower limb and if two ligament complexes are perfectly managed: the tibia-femoral and patello-femoral ligament complexes. From a mathematical point of view, performing a knee joint replacement is therefore a rather complex optimization problem in which the best compromise must be found in order to allow a full range of motion with perfect mobility/stability in both the femoro-patellar as well as the tibio-femoral joint. In this chapter we describe the approach for solving this optimization problem thanks to the integration of several innovative bricks of technology into a so called "Computer Assisted Surgical Protocol", or CASP.

It is worth noting that solutions developed today must be compatible with less invasive surgery; we believe that the recent tendency towards minimally invasive surgery (MIS) in orthopaedics is warranted because it corresponds to a strong need expressed by patients.

In this chapter, we will first describe the CASP specifically developed by Praxim for the LCS knee implant (DePuy Orthopaedics Inc., Warsaw, IN, USA), as well as some novel and innovative bricks of Praxim technology which currently are being integrated into the Surgetics Station (PRAXIM SA, La Tronche, France). The Surgetics Station is an open platform navigation system offering CT-free hip and knee applications that provide geometric AND morphologic 3D data without any preoperative or intraoperative images (no CT, no MR, no fluoroscopy). The method uses data collected intraoperatively with a 3D optical localizer in relative coordinate systems attached to the bones, which is the core Bone Morphing technology (PRAXIM patents pending).

Aims

As in any optimization case, many parameters must be taken into account. None of them are independent and all interact on each other. The main objective for the developer is, firstly, to define a set of goals that must be achieved at the end of the procedure. From a mathematical point of view, these goals will be seen as the output of the optimization loop. Concerning the Praxim CASP developed for the DePuy LCS implant, we wanted to be able to,

- control the alignment of the implants with respect to the mechanical axis, which means to be able to control and plan any tibial and femoral cut in 3D (level and orientation);

- control stability, which requires a soft tissue registration algorithm, under correct alignment;

- manage both soft tissue compartments (femoro-patellar as well as femoro-tibial);

- perform automatic and efficient sizing of the implants;

- perform accurate cuts thanks to intelligent instruments;

- include quality control at each step.

The software relies on 3D geometric and morphologic data. Geometric data may be sufficient for controlling the alignment of the components, but they do not provide a complete representation of the knee. An important drawback of these methods is that they provide only an approximate knee center, by direct digitization or by kinematics analysis of the pathological knee joint, which is rather controversial. Conversely, 3D morphologic data obtained by the bone-morphing technique are very useful to visualize in real time and in three dimensions prior to any real cut: the bone defects, the planned surgical cuts, the choice of the implant size, position and rotation with respect to the bone cortical surfaces, the distances between bones and components. Any of those parameters affects directly the implant position during the planning phase, and all those parameters are linked together.

The Computer-Assisted Surgical Procedure (CASP)

The first step of any CASP is to fix a reference system to each bone or tool we want to track during the surgery. For total knee arthroplasty (TKA), one reference system (DRB) is fixed on the tibia, one on the femur, and one on the patella (optional).

The second step consists of collecting 3D locations of points in order to create the anatomical reference planes (frontal, axial, sagittal) and to build the mechanical axis.

The Center of the Hip

In TKA procedures, the hip is outside the operating field. Therefore, the detection of the center of the joint H is based upon a kinematic method. Once the femoral rigid body is placed, the surgeon performs a circular motion with the lower limb with the knee in full extension. During this motion, the subsequent positions of the femoral rigid body are stored by the computer in the localizer reference system and the center of the hip is calculated.

The Center of the Knee

During TKA procedures, the knee joint is more-or-less open so the digitization of geometric points (landmarks) is relatively easy. Accurate determination of the knee center is difficult because there is no precise definition that applies to the pathological knee. However, the direct localization of an approximation of the center of the pathological knee K_0 is easy using the optical probe. The center is only an indication to compute an approximation of the pathological axes of the patient pre-operatively. In the surgetics approach using bone morphing, the knee center K_p is the center of the knee prosthesis that is planned along each step of the CASP.

The Center of the Ankle

The purely morphological approach that we choose is based on the digitization of two points on the bones. Using the same probe used for the knee joint, the surgeon digitizes one point each on the lateral and medial malleoli. The system computes the middle of the segment defined by these two points. This approach has been extensively investigated and found to be sufficiently accurate and quick to perform.

The Bone Morphing

From the surgical point of view, the bone morphing technique consists of collecting two clouds of points with the probe (one for the femur and one for the tibia). These points are gathered by sliding the spherical tipped probe on the articular surfaces. During this sliding motion, the localizer records the 3D location of the probe tip. This process takes about 1 min 30 for each volume. This point cloud is then matched to a unique deformable model included in the system. The output of this deformation process is an accurate representation of the epiphysis of the bone at surgery. Its accuracy can be checked intraoperatively by the surgeon. The mean error between the model and the actual bone is usually below 0.5 mm.

Morphologic and geometric data will help to optimize the tibial and femoral cuts (location and orientation) in order to solve the complex optimization issue of properly implanting a total knee joint prosthesis (see Fig 10.1 and Fig 10.2).

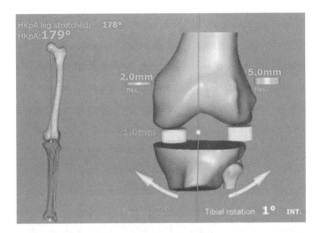

Fig 10.1　Calculated mechanical axis and reconstructed bone surface with morphing technique

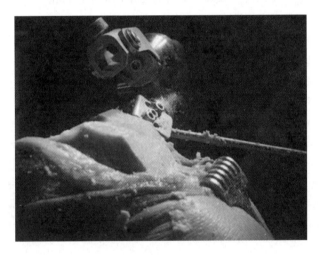

Fig 10.2　Cadaver experiment in open surgery showing femoral cuts milled with the robot

10.2　Principles of MIS in Total Knee Arthroplasty

Introduction

In the past few years, a growing interest has arisen on minimal invasive surgical (MIS) techniques. In orthopedic surgery, in particular, minimally invasive total knee arthroplasty (TKA) has gained special attention. Minimally invasive techniques in joint arthroplasty had, however, a premature birth. In other terms, surgeons have been implanting prosthetic components, already in use and designed without any constraints deriving from the surgical exposure, through reduced skin and soft tissue incisions. Those are either analogous to the traditional ones but smaller or newer and obtained using more innovative approaches and "ad hoc" instruments. MIS technique is, therefore, still evolutionary and this is giving rise to several innovative trends in arthroplasty. Defining MIS technique only based on the incision size is inappropriate: smaller scars should not be the final goal, but only the consequence of a procedure that aims at an increased preservation of the existing and still functional tissues. In total knee arthroplasty, minimally invasive surgery basically means preserving the extensor mechanism. The surgical exposure of the knee joint for bone resection and prosthetic components implantation needs to be performed with the least possible damage to

- the vastus medialis and quadriceps tendon. Von Langebeck's approach, conventionally the most used, involves an incision between tendon and vastus medialis obliquus (VMO) that, after scaring, hinders active contraction and active and passive flexion-extension for a long time. Allowing a patient to undergo a faster rehabilitation and functional recovering is considered one of the most important pillars in MIS TKA;

- the patella and patellar tendon and their blood perfusion. Eversion of the patella stretches the patellar tendon, altering blood perfusion. This induces tendon shortening which can result in a patella baja that is not correlated to unintentional alterations of the joint line.

Three key topics need to be addressed as an overview to MIS TKA.

- The diverse surgical approaches and the instruments enabling them;

- New prosthetic components designed for MIS technique (a field that offers unlimited development opportunities);

- The possibility to combine MIS technique and computer assisted navigation, as a method to control implant alignment and ligament balancing when the surgical approach does not allow a complete and continuous visualization of the joint.

Surgical Techniques

Surgical techniques can be classified into 2 categories: traditional-mini (frontal) and fully innovative techniques (medial and lateral).

The mini midvastus snip and mini-subvastus techniques belong to the first category, whereas the Quad-Sparing technique, in the medial and lateral versions, belongs to the second one. In frontal, midvastus and subvastus, MIS techniques, philosophy and surgical steps are substantially equivalent to those of more traditional approaches.

Minimal invasiveness is reached through surgical approaches designed to preserve tissue and dedicated instruments designed to work in smaller spaces than those available in the past. Fig 10.3 shows a minimally invasive approach to the knee.

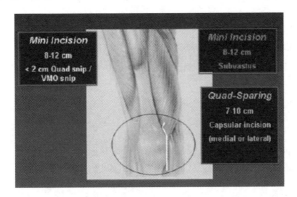

Fig 10.3   Minimally invasive approach to the knee

The quad-sparing technique, instead, brought in true innovation: this new surgical approach avoids any disruption of the vastus medialis obliquus (VMO) — in the medial variant and the vastus lateralis obliquus (VLO) — in the lateral variant throughout the surgical procedure.

All the surgical steps included in the traditional medial and lateral approaches have been modified and the instrument design changes have not only been determined by the reduced incision size but also by the different, i.e. non-frontal, approach.

Patients and Methods

Between June 2003 and December 2005, 52 TKAs were performed with the MIS Quad-Sparing technique using a medial approach and 114 TKAs were performed with the MIS mini-midvastus technique.

The patients suffered from osteoarthritis unresponsive to conservative treatments. TKAs performed in patients with rheumatoid arthritis and revision TKAs are not included in this study.

An important parameter considered in the study was the patient weight, specifically as related to the amount of subcutaneous fat in the distal part of the thigh.

In both patient groups, the same posterior cruciate retaining knee implant model was used.

In the patients operated with the Quad-Sparing technique, the traditionally stemmed plate was substituted with a pegged plate during the first year and with a modular MIS plate during the past year. In the post-operative follow-up, the following parameters have been monitored and evaluated.

● Blood loss in terms of crude loss through the drain in the first 4 hours after surgery, as well as hemoglobin count immediately post-surgery, and in the 1st and in the 3rd day after surgery.

- Range of motion (ROM).
- Implant alignment accuracy, as evaluated by measuring α and β angles on frontal X-ray projections, and γ and σ angles on lateral projections.

Words and Expressions

mechanical axis	力线
lower limb	下肢
ligament complexes	韧带复合体
morphologic [ˌmɔ:fə'lɒdʒɪk]	*adj.* 形态的
cortical surface	皮质表面
tibia ['tɪbɪə]	*n.* 胫骨
femur ['fi:mə]	*n.* 股骨
patella [pə'telə]	*n.* 髌骨
frontal ['frʌntl]	*adj.* 冠状的
axial ['æksɪəl]	*adj.* 横断的，轴线的
sagittal ['sædʒɪtəl]	*adj.* 矢状的
lateral and medial malleoli	外踝和内踝
bone morphing	骨变形
deformable model	变形模型
functional tissue	功能尚存的组织
minimally invasive surgery	微创手术
vastus medialis	股内侧肌
quadriceps tendon	股四头肌腱
flexion-extension	屈伸
rehabilitation [ˌri:həbɪlɪ'teɪʃən]	*n.* 康复
functional recovering	功能恢复
patellar tendon	髌腱
blood perfusion	血液灌注
patella baja	低位髌骨
dedicated instruments	专用仪器
vastus medialis obliquus (VMO)	股内侧斜肌
vastus lateralis obliquus (VLO)	股外侧斜肌
osteoarthritis [ˌɒstɪəʊɑ:'θraɪtɪs]	*n.* 骨关节炎
rheumatoid arthritis	类风湿关节炎
subcutaneous fat	皮下脂肪

post-operative [ˌpəʊstˈɒpərətɪv]   *adj.* 术后的

hemoglobin [ˌhiːməˈɡləʊbɪn]   *n.* 血红蛋白

Key Sentences

1. Both mobility and stability are essential for long term survivorship of the implants and this can only be achieved if the implants are properly aligned with the mechanical axis of the lower limb and if two ligament complexes are perfectly managed: the tibia-femoral and patello-femoral ligament complexes.

参考译文：灵活性和稳定性对于植入物的长期使用至关重要，只有当植入物与下肢的力线准确对齐，并且两个韧带复合体（胫骨–股骨和髌股韧带复合体）得到完美控制时，才能实现这一点。

2. It is worth noting that solutions developed today must be compatible with less invasive surgery; we believe that the recent tendency towards minimally invasive surgery (MIS) in orthopaedics is warranted because it corresponds to a strong need expressed by patients.

参考译文：值得注意的是，如今开发的解决方案必须与微创手术兼容；我们相信，骨科领域最新的微创操作趋势是必然的，因为它呼应了患者的强烈需求。

3. The first step of any CASP is to fix a reference system to each bone or tool we want to track during the surgery. For total knee arthroplasty (TKA), one reference system (DRB) is fixed on the tibia, one on the femur, and one on the patella (optional).

参考译文：对于任何一个 CASP 而言，第一步都要给手术期间待跟踪的各个骨骼或手术器械上固定一个参考系。对于全膝置换手术而言，需要分别在胫骨、股骨、髌骨（可选）上各固定一个参考系（DRB）。

Further Readings

Implications of Minimally Invasive Surgery and CAOS to TKR Design

Introduction

With the recent introduction of MIS and CAOS, an important question is the impact that these new surgical modalities will have on total knee design, and on the short and long-term results. Early experience with smaller incisions with less invasion of muscle tissue has shown advantages in the recovery period, but disadvantages at the time of surgery due to the more limited exposure. In fact, the required space for placing the jigs and fixtures and accessing the saw blades, and the size of present total knee components, places a lower limit on the size of the incision.

Technique

The technique problems can be addressed in a number of ways. Jigs and fixtures can be streamlined and designed to fit the contours of the bones on the medial sides of the femur and tibia. Saw blades can be made narrower with less oscillation displacement, or side-cutting blades or drills could be applied. Using navigation techniques, the direct placement of pins for attaching the slotted cutting guides can eliminate the need for more invasive fixturing and the use of intra-medullary rods. Cutting tools themselves can be navigated, side-stepping the requirement for cutting guides altogether. However, as indicated, the size and shape of the total knee components is not compatible with very small incisions, and often tissue is unduly stretched for access. The possibility is then raised of modifying existing components, or even redesigning completely, to allow for the smallest incisions possible.

Modularizing total knee components is one possibility. For example, the femoral component can be divided either in the sagittal or the frontal planes (see Fig 10.4). The former might be equivalent to a double uni with each uni having a hemi patella flange. The latter might be equivalent to a non-flanged component, with a patella flange added separately. Such schemes can involve split lines over one or more of the bearing surfaces. A sagittal plane split down the center of the patella flange could be acceptable if this area was recessed so that there was no contact with the patella. On the other hand, a transverse split just above the femoro-tibial contact areas, might compromise the patello-femoral bearing in high flexion. If there was a close mechanical join between the modular parts, the problem of fretting would have to be dealt with. Modular components could also be prone to relative movements over time due to differential bone remodeling. In addition, there are stringent alignment requirements at surgery.

Modularization of tibial components may be easier and more sound mechanically. The simplest solutions merely involve a reduction in the depth of the fixation posts rather than modularization. For example, four small posts have shown long-term durability in cemented application for PC-retaining designs (see Fig 10.4). Mini-keels consisting of a shortened central post, with lateral and medial projecting keels of large surface area are already being applied. Although long-term clinical data is not available at this time, theoretical (finite element analysis, FEA) and experimental studies have supported their validity. It is relatively easy to design a modular central post, introduced after the tibial platform has been positioned on the upper tibia. This scheme has the advantage of more closely replicating components which have a long history of successful fixation, but the disadvantages of requiring close tolerances if a taper fit is used, and the requirement of correctly assembling the parts at surgery.

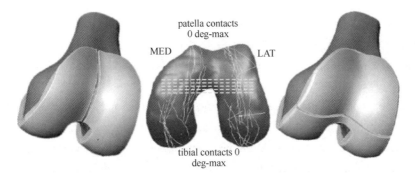

Fig 10.4   Possibilities for modularizing a femoral component for ease of insertion. The central figure shows the paths of the centers of the patello-femoral and femoro-tibial contacts of 6 knee specimens, in the full range of flexion. The dashed area shows the contact region of the patella in the range 120~135 degrees. The sagittally divided femoral component (left) would have not discontinuity of contacts so long as the center of the patella did not contact the bottom of the groove. The frontally divided femoral component (right) would result in a discontinuity of patella tracking in high flexion.

Reducing the size of total knee components to the point of "double unis" with a separate patella flange comprising a set of modular components which can be used selectively for each case, has been advanced by Aubaniac and others. The amount of bone removal is relatively small using such an approach while the existing bone surfaces can be more easily used as templates in order to more accurately restore the original sagittal profiles of the joint, which would especially be beneficial in the sagittal plane from a kinematic point of view. In fixing components to the femur, the use of keels cemented (or uncemented) into slots has proved to be durable. Curved femoral components can even be wrapped around the posterior femur, an advantage for accommodating high flexion. If components for the femur and tibia were housed completely in slots, along the lines of the original polycentric design, surgical preparation of the bone could be greatly simplified. At this time, such a modular component approach may be most appropriate for limited deformity and when both cruciates are preserved. However, it does offer the prospect of achieving more normal function, and it is compatible with small incisions.

Avoiding the use of cement has advantages for small incision surgery. The use of uncemented femoral components has shown similar long-term success as cemented, but there is a requirement for accurate bone preparation and component costs have been higher. On the tibial side, uncemented components have had mixed results, although the use of hydroxyapatite (羟基磷灰石) on metal trays has shown promising results. More recently, composite tibial components have been fabricated, consisting of plastic fused into a trabecular metal backing. Not only has this provided excellent fixation to date, but backside wear is prevented. Notwithstanding the extra costs, enhancements in the surgical precision of bone preparation using CAOS could well lead to a renewal of interest in uncemented components, which could reduce operating time and even extend the duration of the fixation beyond that of cement.

However, a present drawback to using uncemented components is the limited accuracy of using saw blades. It would be an advantage to both improve the accuracy of the bone preparation and the amount of bone removed. This would require a change in the design of the components. On the femoral side, contoured cuts could be made which removed only a few millimeters from the distal femur. To achieve such cuts accurately, several approaches are possible. The first is to use a robotically controlled milling cutter or burring tool, although this would require the acceptance of an active robot. A second approach is a passive robot where the surgeon controls the progress of the cutting tool but where the boundaries are controlled by the robotic arm. The boundaries match the geometry of the implant itself. A third approach, a variant of the passive robot arm, is a cutting tool where the power to the tool is cut off when the tool reaches the prescribed boundaries. Such approaches preferably utilize a burring tool or milling cutter rather than a saw, in which case the volume of bone to be removed should be minimized favoring the curved cuts mentioned above rather than the more traditional square cuts which require much more bone removed. Another way in which bone removal can be reduced for the femoral component is a reduction in the extent of the intercondylar region for the posterior cruciate substituting cam and post. On the tibial side, the bone removal could be reduced by removing primarily those areas beneath the femoral-tibial contact areas, which may also be an advantage to fixation.

Unit 11   Medical Image-Based Disease Prediction

11.1   Computer-Assisted Diagnosis and Radiomics

Introduction

The use and role of medical imaging technologies in clinical oncology has greatly expanded from primarily a diagnostic tool to include a more central role in the context of individualized medicine over the past decade (see Fig 11.1). It is expected that imaging contains complementary and interchangeable information compared to other sources, e.g. demographics, pathology, blood biomarkers, genomics and that combining these sources of information will improve individualized treatment selection and monitoring.

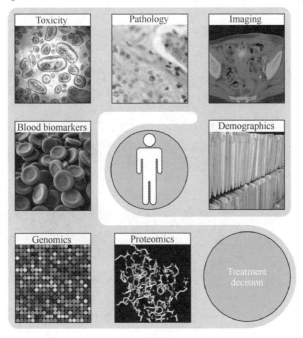

Fig 11.1   Different sources of information, e.g. demographics, imaging, pathology, toxicity, biomarkers, genomics and proteomics, can be used for selecting the optimal treatment

Cancer can be probed in many ways depending on the non-invasive imaging device used or the mode by which it operates. Classically, anatomical computed tomography (CT) imaging is an often-used modality, acquiring images of the "anatome" in high resolution (e.g. 1 mm^3). CT imaging is now routinely used and is playing an essential role in all phases of cancer management, including prediction, screening, biopsy guidance for detection, treatment planning, treatment guidance and treatment response evaluation. CT is used in the assessment of structural features of cancer but it is not perceived to portray functional or molecular details of solid tumours. Functional imaging concerns physiological processes and functions such as diffusion, perfusion and glucose uptake. Here, commonly used methodologies are dynamic contract enhanced-magnetic resonance imaging (DCE-MRI), assessing tumour perfusion and fluoro-2-deoxy-D-glucose (FDG) positron emission tomography (PET) imaging, assessing tumour metabolism, which both often are found to have prognostic value. Finally, another modality is molecular imaging, visualising at the level of specific pathways or macro-molecule in vivo. For example, there are molecular markers assessing tumour hypoxia or labelled antibodies, assessing receptor expression levels of a tumour. Fig 11.2 show the multilevel imaging system.

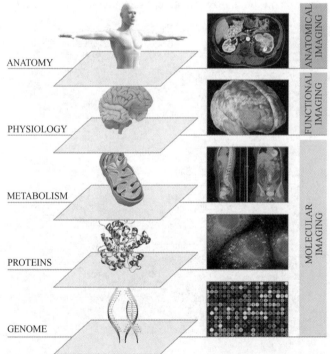

Fig 11.2   Multilevel imaging: anatomical, functional, and molecular imaging

Over the past decades, medical imaging has progressed in four distinct ways.

- Innovations in medical devices (hardware). This concerns improvements in imaging hardware and the development of combined modality machines. For example, in the last decade we moved from single slice CT to multiple slices CT and CT/PET. More recent developments are dual-source and dual-energy CT. These techniques significantly increase the temporal resolution for 4D CT reconstructions allowing visualisation of fine structures in tissues, also in several stages in the cardiac or respiration phase. Moreover, dual-energy CT can be used to improve identification of tissue composition and density.

• Innovations in imaging agents. Innovations in imaging agents (or imaging biomarker, imaging probe, radiotracer), i.e. molecular substances injected in the body and used as an indicator of a specific biological process occurring in the body. This is achieved by contrast agents, i.e. an imaging agent using positive emission tomography (radiotracer). A common use is to find indications of pathological processes, e.g. hypoxia markers using PET imaging.

• Standardised protocol allowing quantitative imaging. Historically, radiology has been a qualitative science, perhaps with the exception of the quantitative use of CT based electron densities in radiotherapy treatment planning. The use of standardised protocols like common MRI spin-echo sequences helps to allow multicentric use of imaging as well as transforming radiology to a more quantitative, highly reproducible science.

• Innovations in imaging analysis. The analysis of medical images has a large impact on the conclusions of the derived images. More and more software is becoming available, allowing for more quantification and standardisation. This has been illustrated by the development of the computer-assisted detection (CAD systems) that improves the performance of detecting cancer in mammography or in lung diseases.

Radiomics focuses on improvements of image analysis, using an automated high-throughput extraction of large amounts (200+) of quantitative features of medical images and belongs to the last category of innovations in medical imaging analysis. The hypothesis is that quantitative analysis of medical image data through automatic or semi-automatic software of a given imaging modality can provide more and better information than that of a physician. This is supported by the fact that patients exhibit differences in tumour shape and texture measurable by different imaging modalities (see Fig 11.3).

The Workflow of Radiomics: A (Semi) High-Throughput Approach

Fig 11.4 depicts the processes involved in the radiomics workflow. The first step involves the acquisition of high quality and standardised imaging, for diagnostic or planning purposes. From this image, the macroscopic tumour is defined, either with an automated segmentation method or alternatively by an experienced radiologist or radiation oncologist. Quantitative imaging features are subsequently extracted from the previously defined tumour region. These features involve descriptors of intensity distribution, spatial relationships between the various intensity levels, texture heterogeneity patterns, descriptors of shape and of the relations of the tumour with the surrounding tissues (i.e. attachment to the pleural wall in lung, differentiation). The extracted image traits are then subjected to a feature selection procedure. The most informative features are identified based on their independence from other traits, reproducibility and prominence on the data. The selected features are then analysed for their relationship with treatment outcomes or gene expression. The ultimate goal is to provide accurate risk stratification by incorporating the imaging traits into predictive models for treatment outcome and to evaluate their added value to commonly used predictors.

（a）　　　　　　　（b）　　　　　　　（c）

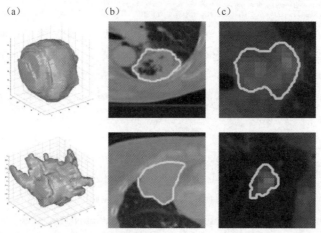

Fig 11.3　(a) Two representative 3D representations of a round tumour (top) and spiky tumour (bottom) measured by computed tomography (CT) imaging. (b) Texture differences between non-small cell lung cancer (NSCLC) tumours measured using CT imaging, more heterogeneous (top) and more homogeneous (bottom). (c) Differences of FDG-PET uptake, showing heterogeneous uptake

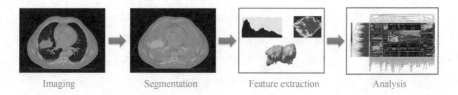

Imaging　　　　　Segmentation　　　Feature extraction　　　Analysis

Fig 11.4　The radiomics workflow

11.2　Medical Image-Based Alzheimer Disease Prediction

Introduction

Alzheimer's disease (AD) is the most common neurodegenerative dementia, which

causes the gradual loss of cognitive functions. A definite diagnosis of AD can only be made through autopsy findings, such as amyloid deposition and neurofibrillary tangles. In practice, the diagnosis of AD is based on clinical criteria. In addition, findings from neuroimaging technologies, such as magnetic resonance imaging (MRI), positron emission tomography (PET), or single-photon emission computed tomography could further increase the diagnostic accuracy of AD. Among these modalities, structural MRI has been recognized as a marker for neuronal injury, which could be detected as volume loss, cortical thinning, or changes in shape seen in a set of anatomical structures such as the medial temporal area, the posterior cingulate area, the thalamus, and other cortical areas.

One promising extension of these findings in anatomical MRI is the use in the analysis of large clinical data, in which a large number of anatomical MRIs of an elderly population, collected through multiple institutes, could be used to evaluate the possibility of AD or to evaluate the future risk for developing dementia, on an individual basis. A range of studies have demonstrated that morphometric features extracted from structural MRI, along with machine-learning techniques, could be used to classify a single subject as a member of a particular clinical category. One group of these studies considers voxel-based tissue probability maps directly as features in the classification. Another group focuses on regional characteristics, such as volume, shape, thickness within one single anatomical structure, or the multivariate description over the whole-brain parcels obtained using automated segmentation tools. The third group first characterizes the shape of an ROI as a series of parameters, such as spherical harmonics or log-Jacobian determinants from tensor-based morphometry, and then utilizes the parameters as features. Some other studies have focused on the combination of multiple modalities, including MRI, PET, and cerebrospinal fluid (CSF), and have yielded good classification accuracies.

In a previous study, a residual-based measurement using an atlas grid was reported, which could successfully capture anatomical features of various types of neurodegenerative diseases. This approach was named the Gross feature recognition of Anatomical Images based on Atlas grid (GAIA), which is a highly time-efficient method for the image recognition and does not rely on non-linear transformation. In this approach, an atlas with more than 200 pre-defined structures was linearly superimposed on a target image and the intensities of the defined structures were measured. The intensity rankings of the defined structures were then used as anatomical features. Anatomical alterations beyond the normal range would lead to gross misregistration and abnormal intensities of the defined structures, which was captured as an anatomical feature. Although utilization of the pre-defined atlas grid (i.e. anatomical structure parcellation map) is an effective way for dimensional reduction, one of the limitations of GAIA is reduced sensitivity to localized anatomical alterations that only affect part of a pre-defined structure.

In our study, we extended the GAIA approach to voxel-based feature recognition, in which, instead of applying a pre-defined atlas grid for feature extraction and reduction, we employed data-specific and knowledge-based masks. These masks were created based on voxel-based statistics results and the Disease-Specific Anatomical Filtering method. Because GAIA relies on image intensities, standardization of voxel intensity values across different images is one of the technical challenges. To standardize the intensity of MRI images, histogram equalization, in which the tonal distribution of an input image and a template are mathematically matched, is often used. However, the spatial relationship between pixels in the target image and the template is disregarded in this approach, which sometimes leads to artifacts caused by the increased contrast-to-noise ratio in low-intensity areas. Therefore, for voxel-based analysis, we introduced the local binary pattern (LBP), which has been widely used in various applications and has been proven robust to monotonic gray-level changes, and is also computationally efficient. A frequent application of LBP is facial recognition attributed to its invariance to illumination changes in facial pictures. Similarly, cross-scanner variability in MRI images can also be characterized as a monotonic change, where the ranking value of the average intensity in a particular anatomical tissue would not change over subjects. For instance, in T1-weighted images, the intensities of gray matter pixels are always lower than those of white matter pixels in an image retrieved from any scanner.

Method

Preprocessing

The structural MRI images were first skull-stripped using a Matlab suite called SPM8. To be specific, a brain mask was obtained for each subject by combining three individual tissue probability maps, including white matter, gray matter, and cerebrospinal fluid (CSF), obtained from the unified segmentation module incorporated in SPM. The mask was then superimposed on the original image to clean up tissues outside the brain, such as the skull, skin, and neck. Skull-stripped images were then co-registered (linear transformed) to a template, namely EVE, using 12 degrees of freedom (DOF) affine to standardize each individual to the Montreal Neurological Institute (MNI) space. To obtain an unbiased co-registration, 12 degrees of freedom affine were employed with cost function setting to mutual information (MI), which was proved robust to inter-subject intensity variations. After the co-registration, spatial locations and global brain sizes, which were considered as covariates in analyzing the disease-specific features, were normalized for all these subjects.

Gray-Level Invariant Features

LBP operator was used to represent the gray-level invariant features of the original image with low computational complexity. It described the local structure by thresholding the intensities of a set of P neighboring pixels set (IP) with the intensity of its center pixel IC, and then represented the feature as a binary code, as explained in Eq.(11.1). A demonstration of its gray-level invariance is shown in Fig 11.5, where LBP is applied to 2D phantom MRIs with multiple monotonic gray-level changes. MRI images shown in the first row of Fig 11.5 were simulated by BrainWeb by setting the simulated Flip Angle to 10, 20, and 40 respectively. The second row shows corresponding LBP maps, which, as expected, differed little from each other. The reason for using phantom images is to guarantee that all images were exactly in the same coordinate.

$$\text{LBP} = \sum_{p=0}^{p-1} \text{sign}(I_p - I_c)2^p, \quad \text{sign}(x) = \begin{cases} 1, & x \geq 0 \\ 0, & x < 0 \end{cases} \tag{11.1}$$

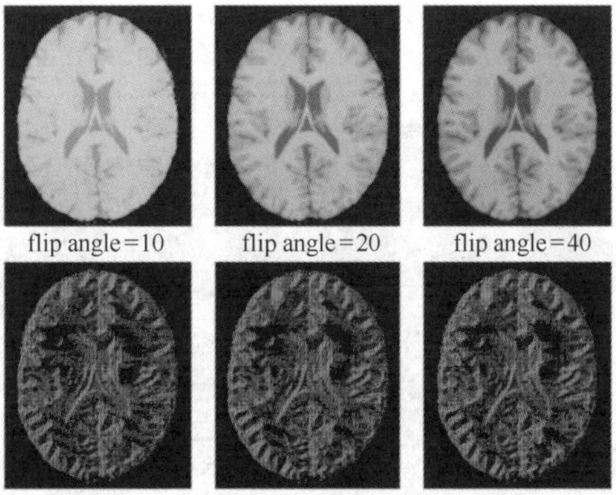

flip angle=10   flip angle=20   flip angle=40

Fig 11.5   A 2D LBP test on simulated MRIs. The first row displays the MRI images and the second row displays their corresponding LBP maps. Images scanned with different flip angles are shown in columns

Rotation invariant LBP was an extended version of the original operator with robustness to image rotation. Given that affine has been applied to exclude the rotation influence, traditional LBP operator was deemed competent for feature extraction in the present study, which resulted in 256 possible labels within a 363 neighborhood. In this case, the intensity of the LBP map ranged from 0 to 255 in a 2D image. A straightforward 3D LBP form, namely LBP-TOP (three orthogonal planes), was proposed in a previous study to describe spatiotemporal signals of facial expression by simply concatenating features extracted from three orthogonal 2D planes. In the present study, LBP-TOP operator traversed all 363 neighborhoods in every 2D slice varying separately along axial, coronal, and sagittal orientations, as shown in Fig 11.6. Thus, every pixel P was potentially represented by a 3D vector [LBP$_{xP}$ LBP$_{yP}$ LBP$_{zP}$], denoting the LBP value separately on the y-z, x-z, and x-y planes. The 3D vector was used as image features for Alzheimer's disease diagnosis.

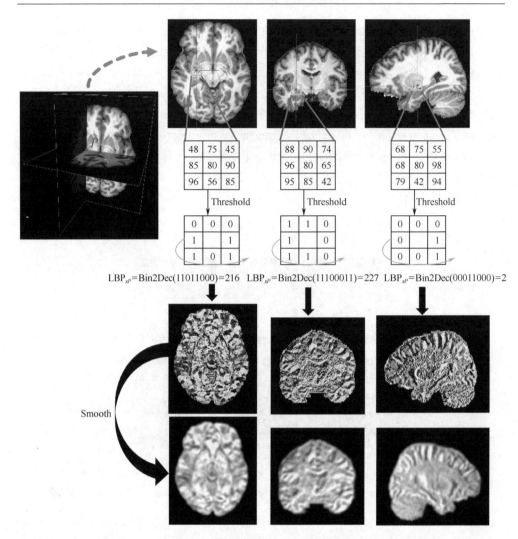

Fig 11.6　A brief illustration of the calculation of LBP-TOP value in pixel P in the axial, coronal, and sagittal orientations. Pixel P is denoted by the red color, with its 363 neighborhoods circled by a yellow square in the 2D plane. Bin2Dec is a function for transferring binary code to decimal values

Words and Expressions

radiomics	*n.* 影像组学
individualized medicine	个体化医疗，个体化医学
complementary [ˌkɒmplɪ'mentəri]	*adj.* 互补的，补充的
interchangeable[ˌɪntə'tʃeɪndʒəbəl]	*adj.* 可交换的，可互换的

demographics [ˌdeməˈɡræfiks]	*n.* 人口统计学
pathology [pəˈθɒlədʒi]	*n.* 病理学
blood biomarker	血液生物标志物
genomics [dʒəˈnəʊmɪks]	*n.* 基因组学
treatment response evaluation	治疗反应评估
physiological process	生理过程
glucose uptake	葡萄糖摄取
metabolism [məˈtæbəlɪzəm]	*n.* 新陈代谢
molecular imaging	分子成像
tumour hypoxia	肿瘤缺氧
antibody [ˈæntɪˌbɒdi]	*n.* 抗体
receptor expression level	受体表达水平
dual-source and dual-energy CT	双源双能 CT
temporal resolution	时间分辨率
cardiac or respiration phase	心脏或呼吸周期
imaging agent	显像剂
radiotracer [ˈreɪdɪəʊtreɪsə]	*n.* 放射性示踪剂
pathological processes	病理过程
radiotherapy [ˌreɪdɪəʊˈθerəpi]	*n.* 放射治疗
pleural wall	胸膜壁
informative [ɪnˈfɔːmətɪv]	*adj.* 提供有用信息的
reproducibility [ˌriːprəˌdjuːsɪˈbɪlɪti]	*n.* 可重复性
risk stratification	危险分层
Alzheimer's disease	阿尔茨海默病
neurodegenerative dementia	神经退行性痴呆
cognitive function	认知功能
morphometric	*adj.* 形态测量的
covariate [ˌkʌˈveəriət]	*n.* 协变量
orthogonal [ɔːˈθɒɡənəl]	*adj.* 正交的

Key Sentences

1. The use and role of medical imaging technologies in clinical oncology has greatly expanded from primarily a diagnostic tool to include a more central role in the context of individualized medicine over the past decade.

参考译文： 在过去的十年里，医学影像技术在临床肿瘤学中的应用和作用已经从最初的诊断工具扩展到在个体化医学背景下的核心工具。

2. CT imaging is now routinely used and is playing an essential role in all phases of cancer management, including prediction, screening, biopsy guidance for detection, treatment planning, treatment guidance and treatment response evaluation.

参考译文：目前，CT 成像已被常规应用于临床，并在癌症治疗的所有阶段都发挥着重要作用，包括预测、筛查、引导活检检查、制订治疗计划、提供治疗指导和评估治疗反应等。

3. To obtain an unbiased co-registration, 12 degrees of freedom affine were employed with cost function setting to mutual information (MI), which was proved robust to inter-subject intensity variations.

参考译文：为了实现无偏的配准，将采用 12 自由度仿射，其中成本函数基于互信息（MI），这种方法被证明对受试者之间的强度变化具有较高的健壮性。

Further Readings

Mammographic Image-Based Breast Cancer Prediction

Since the majority of breast cancers are detected in women without known risk factors, a uniformly applied mammography screening protocol is currently recommended for all women who qualify for screening (e.g. annual screening for women over 40 years old in the United States). Early detection combined with improved treatment strategies have incrementally and significantly reduced patients' mortality and morbidity rates over the last four decades. However, interpreting mammograms is a difficult and time-consuming task in a screening environment due to large variability in the depicted breast abnormalities, overlapping dense fibroglandular tissue, and low cancer prevalence (i.e. 3~5 cancers in 1,000 non-baseline screening examinations). These factors substantially reduce detection sensitivity and specificity of mammography, in particular in younger women with dense breast tissue as well as in other high-risk groups. The specificity of mammography is also low. One study reported that during a 10-year period, more than half of screened women would receive at least one false-positive recall and 7% ~ 9% would have at least one benign biopsy. In addition to women's anxiety, which can cause long-term psychosocial consequences, and potential harmful effects due to cumulative radiation exposure and unnecessary biopsies, limited health care resources and associated high costs are also issues that will have to be addressed in current breast cancer screening practices. As a result, the efficacy of current mammography screening remains quite controversial. To overcome the limitations of current population-based mammography screening practices, it is desirable to make personalized screening recommendations based on individualized risk assessment, and this concept has been recently attracting significant research interest. The ultimate goal of developing and implementing a personalized cancer screening paradigm is to enable the identification of a small fraction of women with significantly higher than average near-term risk of developing breast cancer. As a result, this small fraction of high-risk women should be more frequently screened (e.g. annually or perhaps even more frequently), while the vast majority of women at average or lower risk of developing cancer in the near-term could be screened at longer intervals (e.g. every 2~5 years) until their near-term cancer risk has significantly increased.

In our group, we have preliminarily investigated a computerized method to detect bilateral mammographic density asymmetry between left and right breasts, and the potential of using the computed bilateral mammographic density asymmetry scores to predict the risk of a woman developing breast cancer after a negative screening examination of interest. In this study, we aim to assess the feasibility of applying a machine learning method to develop a near-term breast cancer risk prediction model using an expanded image dataset and a new analytical method. Our hypothesis is that the bilateral mammographic tissue or density asymmetry between the left and right breasts is an important radiographic image phenotype related to abnormal biologic processes that may lead to cancer development, and an increase in bilateral mammographic density asymmetry could be an important indicator of developing breast abnormality or cancer. As an example, Fig 11.7 shows four sets of bilateral mammograms acquired from two women during two repeated (sequential) screening examinations. The "baseline" examinations of interest were interpreted clinically as "negative" by the radiologists. During the next subsequent examination, cancer was detected in the woman showing a higher degree of bilateral mammographic density asymmetry on the baseline examination, while the other woman remained "negative" although she had overall higher but more symmetrically mammographic density on the baseline examination. However, subjectively rating mammographic density is difficult and inconsistent due to the large intra- and interobserver variability. Since studies have demonstrated that using a computerized scheme enabled achievement of more consistent results in assessing mammographic tissue density on individual images, we will also develop and apply a computerized scheme to detect bilateral mammographic tissue or density asymmetry.

The negative "baseline" bilateral CC view images (left) are shown side-by-side with the corresponding subsequent mammogram (right). The woman whose images are displayed on the top row was diagnosed as having invasive mammary carcinoma (arrow) in the subsequent examination while the one displayed on the bottom row remained negative.

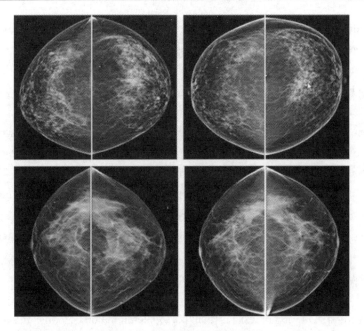

Fig 11.7　An example of bilateral mammographic density asymmetry of a positive and a negative case

In this study, we built an artificial neural network (ANN) on the basis of a set of image features computed from negative digital mammograms prior to the detection of the abnormalities in question, in order to generate a new classification score that represents bilateral mammographic density asymmetry. We then applied the ANN-generated bilateral mammographic density asymmetry scores to predict the likelihood of a woman developing a "detectable" breast cancer or a high-risk lesion on the subsequent mammographic screening examination acquired between 12 and 36 months following the negative screening examination of interest.

Method

We first applied a computerized scheme that uses an iterative threshold method to segment breast area from the air background depicted on each CC (craniocaudal) view image, and then computed five mammographic tissue composition and density related image features using previously reported methods directly from the original FFDM images. In brief, these include four-pixel value based statistical features, namely (a) mean pixel value of the whole segmented breast area depicted on one image, (b) standard deviation, (c) skewness and (d) kurtosis of all pixel values. The fifth feature represents the local variation (or local maximum difference in pixel values) within a region of interest (R) with a radius r. For each pixel (x, y) inside the breast area, the local variation is $V(x, y, R) = \max_{(i,j) \in R} I(i, j) - \min_{(i,j) \in R} I(i, j)$, whereby (i, j) is the coordinate of the neighboring pixel. The total local variation as the function of r is computed as $V(r) = \sum\limits_{(x,y) \in R} V(x,y,R(r))$. Then, the scheme estimates fractal dimension (FD) from the relationship $V(r) \propto r^{2-FD}$ by fitting a straight line to the $V(r)$ versus r function. The slope of the fitted line is used as the fifth image feature. The computerized scheme was independently applied to each CC view image of the left and right breasts in order to segment the breast area and compute the five image features. Finally, five feature differences were computed by subtracting matched features computed from the two bilateral CC view images, $\Delta F_i = |F_i^L - F_i^R|$, where $i = 1, 2, \cdots, 5$. To generate the bilateral mammographic density asymmetry score by combining these five computed image feature differences, we built a simple three-layer ANN. The ANN has five input neurons (represented by the five computed image feature differences) in the first (input) layer, two hidden neurons in the second layer, and one decision neuron in the third (output) layer. To minimize the training/testing bias when using the ANN, we used a leave-one-case-out (LOCO) method to compute and obtain a bilateral mammographic density asymmetry score for each case in our testing dataset. For example, when we compared the risk prediction performance between the 230 positive and 230 negative cases (total 460 cases), the ANN was first trained using 459 cases, and the trained ANN was then applied to the one remaining (left out) case to obtain a bilateral mammographic density asymmetry score (ranging from 0 to 1). The higher the score, the higher the bilateral mammographic density asymmetry level is. This process was repeated 460 times, whereby each case was used in the training sample in 459 cycles and as a test sample once. The same ANN training/testing protocol reported and used in our previous study was applied in all 460 training/testing computations. The LOCO method was also applied to train and test the other two sets of ANNs for classification between the positive and benign cases as well as between the benign and negative cases.

Unit 12　Human Factors Engineering: Design of Medical Devices

12.1　Introduction of Human Factors Engineering

Human factors engineering (HFE) is the application of knowledge about human capabilities (physical, sensory, emotional, and intellectual) and limitations to the design and development of tools, devices, systems, environments, and organizations. HFE might also be called human factors, ergonomics, human engineering, usability engineering, or human-computer interaction (HCI). HFE involves the use of behavioral science and engineering methodologies in support of design and evaluation.

Successful development of safe and usable medical devices and systems requires the application of HFE principles and processes throughout the product design cycle. Doing so can help reduce use error, enhance patient and user safety, improve product usability and efficiency, and enhance user satisfaction. The relationship between HFE and risk management in reducing use error is addressed in International Electrotechnical Commission (IEC) 62366:2007, Medical devices—Application of usability engineering to medical devices.

Many decades of basic and applied research, as well as practical experience, have generated a substantial base of scientific knowledge about people and their interactions with each other, with technology, and with their environment. For example, extensive data are available on the size and shape of the human body (anthropometry), how people sense the world (perception), how people think (cognition), and how they act (sensory/motor performance). These data and related principles governing their application are available in numerous textbooks, technical articles, standards and guidelines, and specialized design tools. Knowledge of HFE methods and principles is critical to the design of safe and effective medical devices. It allows device designers to choose wisely among design alternatives. It also allows designers to validate that a design is appropriate for use in a clinical context. HFE areas of special importance relate to understanding the factors that affect human performance, the nature of human error and human fallibility, the role of humans in complex systems, and the causes of use errors (e.g. inadvertent control activation). The HFE process for medical device design and evaluation is discussed in detail in ANSI/AAMI HE74:2001

(R2009), Human factors design process for medical devices, and in comparable international standards. HFE is not blind adherence to a set of guidelines.

12.2   HFE Medical Device Design

Although an understanding of detailed human factors guidelines is helpful when designing a medical device, a command of the general principles — what some people might informally call "rules of thumb" — is critical. After all, clinicians and users can usually cope with devices that have specific design shortcomings, provided that the flaws do not lead to serious use errors or pose insurmountable obstacles to accomplishing a task. In fact, few device-user interface designs are perfect; they usually violate one specific guideline or another. It can be much more serious if a medical device violates a general human factors design principle.

Serious violations, such as presenting information too quickly or expecting users to carefully read a manual before using a device, can render a medical device unsafe and unusable. Designers should focus on meeting the high-level design principles before they perfect the details. After all, there is no sense in refining a fundamentally flawed product. In contrast, great products arise from fundamentally correct solutions that are then honed to a state of excellence.

This section presents several high-level design principles intended to help designers produce fundamentally correct user interfaces.

12.2.1   Seek User Input

Involve Users Early and Often

Users can offer invaluable guidance at several stages of user-interface development. Early in the design process, users can critique existing devices, offer a vision of optimal interactions with the medical device, and help set usability objectives. As an interface design evolves, testing can identify design characteristics that users like or dislike and, more importantly, that are difficult to use or cause use errors. Toward the end of the design process, users can help verify near-final designs by participating in usability testing of working prototypes. Thus, user involvement throughout the design process helps to ensure that the final device meets its intended users' actual needs. It also avoids last-minute design modifications to address unanticipated usability problems, which can be quite expensive and which might not be entirely effective.

Refine Designs Through Usability Testing

Usability testing is arguably the cornerstone of the human factors engineering process. It is good business to thoroughly evaluate a device's user interface before commercial deployment, when use error can put patients and users at risk. Progressive manufacturers might choose to extend testing beyond primary tasks (e.g. using a defibrillator to shock a patient in cardiac arrest) and documentation to include setup, storage, maintenance, and even repair tasks.

Usability testing is a well-established method of discerning user-interface design issues that could affect safety, efficacy, and satisfaction. In a typical test session, representative device users perform targeted tasks in an appropriate environment, which could range from a conference room to a sophisticated, high-fidelity simulation of the intended clinical care environment. The level of test fidelity usually increases as the device progresses from a concept to a refined prototype. Testing early in the design process and then several more times as the design evolves is an effective way to prevent user interaction problems from persisting into the later stages of the design process, when effective solutions to problems are more limited and more expensive to implement.

Test administrators should take particular care when choosing test participants. It is important to find a sample of participants who accurately reflect the range of user characteristics — rather than, for example, choosing "thought leaders" who bring special knowledge and motivation to the test. User characteristics that should be considered include physical attributes (i.e. ergonomics), abilities and skills, needs, and psychological attributes.

12.2.2　Establish Design Priorities

Keep It Simple

In medical device design, simpler is usually better. Most users dislike devices equipped with all the "bells and whistles", especially if the "extras" get in the way of performing basic tasks. Indeed, some medical devices are loaded with features intended to give the products a competitive advantage against competing products. Yet, features aimed at enhancing sales can cost a company customer goodwill if they complicate device operation. Accordingly, designers are well served to produce devices that focus on the basics and exclude features offering little day-to-day value. Adding complexity for "bells and whistles" that interfere with initial ease of use is usually not worth it. That said, designers should be careful about eliminating advanced features that offer real value to sophisticated users, even if such users are a small percentage of the user base. In such cases, faced with divergent market needs, manufacturers should consider developing two products rather than a single, compromised version.That is to say, different devices should be manufactured for different use populations (see Fig 12.1). Ultrasound scanners from different manufacturers are targeted toward different user populations and use environments. The scanner on the left is intended for highly mobile use by less sophisticated users than the one on the right. Similarly, designers should seek ways to limit the level of skill needed to maintain and repair a device, as well as the number of steps and the need for special tools.

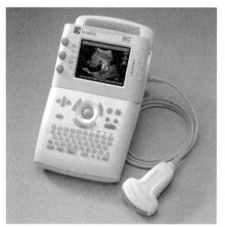 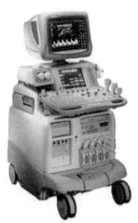

Fig 12.1   Different devices for different use populations

Ensure Safe Use

Medical devices should minimize the risk of injury (both physical and psychological) to users or patients during normal and emergency use. Applying this principle to a computed tomography (CT) scanner, designers should promote design solutions that reduce users' risk of trauma from moving parts and that prevent patients from feeling claustrophobic because of being enclosed in a tight space. Applying the principle to a portable patient monitor, designers should avoid placing a heavy instrument on a wheeled pole that is vulnerable to tip over, an outcome that could injure both clinicians and patients, cause property damage, and disrupt the care delivery process. Designers should also consider the consequences of dynamic user interactions. For example, a portable glucose monitor for home use should be designed so that the control-display relationships minimize the risk of the diabetic user (who could have a dangerously low blood sugar) collecting the sample incorrectly or misreading the resulting value. Thus, potential device-induced harm can result from static design characteristics (i.e. the physical design can have mechanical consequences) or from use errors during device interaction.

Fig 12.2 is an example of a portable device configured for safety and usability. To enhance mobility, safety, and convenience when responding to a medical emergency, a defibrillator, oxygen bottle, and intravenous (IV) pole are mounted on a stable cart.

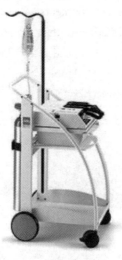

Fig 12.2　Portable device configured for safety and usability

Ensure Essential Communication

During busy and stressful moments, people must work harder to communicate with each other, which might lead them to raise their voices, repeat themselves to make sure they are heard, or even grasp someone's arm to get their attention. Similarly, a well-designed medical device should be capable of reliably communicating critical information, such as a life-threatening change in a patient's vital signs, during busy and stressful moments. To do so, the device probably needs a sufficiently loud auditory alarm signal to complement a visual alarm signal, thereby using two sensory channels to increase the chance of detection. Moreover, the visual alarm signal might flash to draw attention and the auditory alarm signal might be set at an attention-getting frequency.

Accordingly, devices should employ redundant methods of communicating vital information. Also, when possible, devices should provide users with a clear and concise explanation of any problem (including the source) and how to correct it. Finally, all designs should be evaluated in the context of the overall use environment, including other devices commonly used there, to ensure that the design solution does not result in unintended consequences, including impaired clinician-patient, clinician-clinician, or clinician-device communication.

Anticipate Device Failures

Devices will fail. When they do, it is important to communicate the failure to users and, when possible, indicate the cause and recommended remedial actions. Such communication is especially important if a failure places a patient at immediate risk (e.g. failure of an air-in-blood detector). Ideally, devices should fail safely, but human intervention might be needed to ensure a safe outcome.

Therefore, designers should consider the full range of device failure modes (including use errors) and develop strategies and detailed user interfaces or other solutions for coping with them, including dynamic enunciation of anticipated failure modes with suggested prevention or mitigation strategies. The cause of the failure and proper remedial or coping actions should be communicated clearly and concisely.

Facilitate Workflow

Humans are resistant to change. Users will be reluctant to learn and to use a new medical device (or new device model) unless they appreciate a real payoff in terms of work efficiency or effectiveness. Therefore, designers should understand how their device could affect the user and the task environment, including task information flow and user workload. Analysis of how people will use the device will help designers organize the user interface to facilitate urgent, frequent, and critical tasks. For example, designers might want to provide a dedicated, surface-level control for recording a physiological waveform rather than relegate the control to a lower-level software screen. Potential device uses should be formally analyzed using techniques such as contextual inquiry, task analysis, or usability testing.

12.2.3   Accommodate User Characteristics and Capabilities

Do Not Expect Users to Become Masters

Most users master only the device's critical (from their perspective) features, even if the device is only modestly complex. A comparison of varying levels of mastery of infusion pump tasks is shown in Table 12.1. In other words, practical-minded and time-pressed users master just the features that they use frequently. Users tend to disregard other device features until they are forced to deal with them, expecting at that time to draw on their experience, intuition and peer support to operate the device correctly. Accordingly, designers should make infrequently performed tasks particularly intuitive (especially if the task is life-critical) because most users will approach them in the same manner as novices.

Table 12.1 Comparison of varying levels of mastery of infusion pump tasks

Sample user	Level of mastery of performing specific tasks		
	Determine the total volume of IV fluid infused	Set up a "piggyback" infusion	Change the battery
Nurse X	High	Medium	Low
Physician Y	Medium	Low	Low
Biomedical Engineer Z	Medium	Low	High

Expect Use Errors

Many things contribute to device use error. Therefore, while maintaining a respectful view of users, designers should assume that users will make errors. They should not assume that all users will operate a device with equivalent levels of preparation, attitude, vigilance, or motivation. Instead, a disconcerting proportion of users might have insufficient training, might have forgotten their training since last using the device, might have insufficient aptitude for interacting with technology, might become fatigued from working long hours, or might be rushing or distracted by other tasks. Designers should overestimate, rather than underestimate, the chances of use errors. Thus, designers should make the errors obvious to users, provide for rapid error recovery, and guide users through the recovery process. For example, if the user inadvertently types in the wrong dose of drug to be administered (e.g. the user hits the 7 key instead of the 1 key and an excessive dose is specified), the infusion device's software could indicate that the resulting dose is greater than that allowed by the hospital for this drug and then provide the acceptable dose range.

Accommodate Diverse Users

It is perilous for designers to assume that user populations are homogeneous. All users are not just like them. Many human factors researchers conduct fieldwork leading to the formulation of user profiles of typical as well as extreme users that can help to guide the design effort. Some devices have small and specialized populations of users, such as highly trained interventional cardiologists who operate catheterization laboratory equipment. In contrast, over-the-counter devices, such as glucose meters, blood pressure monitors, metered dose inhalers, and infant apnea monitors, are used by quite diverse individuals, including the young, the old, and people with disabilities (see Fig 12.3). Designs should accommodate the needs of users who have different sizes, shapes, physical abilities, intellectual capabilities, and experiences. A simple example of accommodating user diversity is the design of a surgical tool that can be used comfortably by individuals with either small or large hands.

Other examples include a patient data entry screen used by people who have extensive computer experience as well as those with relatively little experience, or a mammography machine that is usable by both healthy individuals and those in wheelchairs.

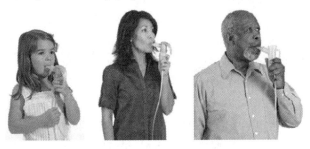

Fig 12.3   Device users of varying ages

Maximize Accessibility

The term "accessibility" has traditionally been associated with architectural features, such as sidewalks, building entrances, and restrooms. Features such as curb cuts, automatic doors, and restroom stalls equipped with assist bars are products of regulations and political activism that have improved accessibility to public spaces. In recent years, consumer electronic and information technology products have incorporated features that make them more accessible to users with physical or sensory impairments. For example, U.S. government websites now describe all figures in the text. Medical devices can be improved similarly to make them more usable for people with a wide range of cognitive, perceptual, and physical disabilities. Devices will be made more accessible to such users if they are considered when designers are establishing user requirements and then designing to those requirements. An example of an accessible therapeutic device is a glucose meter that provides directions and meter readings verbally to facilitate use by individuals with visual impairments. Fig 12.4 depicts a personal emergency pendant communicator which allows communication with the push of a button.

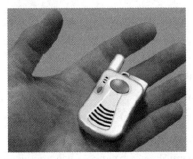

Fig 12.4   A personal emergency pendant communicator

Consider External Factors That Influence Task Performance

Sometimes, people use medical devices in a relatively isolated manner (e.g. a user reprograms an insulin pump while seated at a desk in a quiet room). However, people often use medical devices in more distracting settings that could be quite noisy or particularly hot (e.g. outdoor settings or ambulances on hot days). Other people near the medical device could be vying for the user's attention. Users might have to split their attention among several devices or could be wearing protective gear (e.g. glasses and gloves) to prevent contamination or injury. Designers who consider these and other external factors might learn that a design is incompatible with some uses. For example, a paramedic might find it difficult to press a button while wearing thick gloves or to read a display at an acute angle. Also, some devices might be used in very constrained spaces (see Fig 12.5).

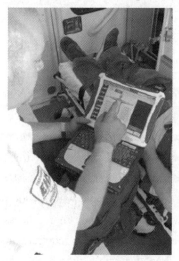

Fig 12.5　Devices used in very constrained spaces

12.2.4　Accommodate Users' Needs and Preferences

Prioritize User Input

Medical device users, particularly at large hospitals that purchase large numbers of devices, often ask manufacturers to customize devices according to their institutions' needs. Such requests might motivate designers to design configuration options for devices. This approach supports the appropriate goal of making devices adapt to the users, rather than the other way around. However, such adaptability could make user interfaces less stable or less predictable and even compromise performance. Users accustomed to one device could be confused when they encounter a similar device with a completely different setup. For example, a nurse who works at several different hospitals each week might encounter infusion pumps that look the same but work quite differently, setting the stage for use errors because of negative transference. One solution is to limit user-interface variability by developing optimal solutions for all users (when possible) and then making the remaining interface differences obvious. This approach might be resisted, however, because it asks manufacturers to sacrifice brand identity and competitive advantages in favor of commonality.

Manufacturer compliance with de facto industry standards might be compromised by existing patents and licensing agreements. An alternative is to design a device that can be readily set to a particular institution's or individual's preferences, thereby accommodating market niches, while ensuring that such preferences do not impede typical users. Finally, designers should remember that although users might express specific needs and preferences — or even suggest a detailed design — their suggestions might prove unworkable, undesirable, or unreliable. Designers should act as interpreters, taking and prioritizing input from users while also applying their own expertise and creativity to produce the best possible designs.

When interface design tradeoffs (e.g. better brand identity vs. potentially improved usability by conforming to industry conventions or user expectations) are made explicit, empirical testing (i.e. functional usability testing) can be performed to better inform corporate decisions.

Do Not Rely Exclusively on "Thought Leaders"

It can be tempting to rely on guidance from accomplished clinicians or clinician technophiles, sometimes referred to as "thought leaders". However, such individuals might not use the pertinent technology regularly. Similarly, there might be pressure to rely on individuals who represent large accounts, the goal being to give extra emphasis to those particular institutions' needs in order to retain their business. Indeed, such individuals can be an excellent source of design input, particularly with regard to identifying user needs and preferences. However, thought leaders and existing clients might have a relatively more sophisticated viewpoint as well as more extensive knowledge of device-specific design issues and tradeoffs. Also, such individuals might push a particular design solution harder than appropriate because of preconceived biases or an emotional investment. Finally, existing customers who are familiar with predecessor devices might bias designs away from design improvements that would actually improve device performance but represent new hardware investment and retraining. Accordingly, design teams should seek input from a wide variety of users who are appropriately representative of typical intended users.

Let Users Set the Pace

Human beings generally become annoyed when machines set the work pace. It is inevitable that the pace will be too slow or too fast, owing to individual performance differences as well as differences over time (e.g. changes in performance because of fatigue). Moreover, machine-paced tasks do not always allow for work stoppages or interruptions (e.g. emergency situations). Thus, humans tend to prefer to feel that they are "in control" of processes and technology. Designers should let users set the work pace (e.g. by requiring them to provide a confirmation of task completion before proceeding to the next step in a procedure).

Words and Expressions

human factors engineering	人机工程学，人因工程学
ergonomics [ˌɜːgəˈnɒmɪks]	n. 工效学
human-computer interaction	人机交互
International Electrotechnical Commission	国际电工委员会
anthropometry [ˌænθrəˈpɒmɪtrɪ]	n. 人体测量，人体测量学
perception [pəˈsepʃən]	n. 知觉，感知
cognition [kɒgˈnɪʃən]	n. 认知，感知，认识
human error	人为失误
fallibility [ˌfæləˈbɪləti]	n. 易错性，不可靠性
rule of thumb	经验法则，拇指规则，经验原则
working prototype	原型机
defibrillator [diːˈfɪbrəleɪtə]	n. 除颤器
cardiac arrest	心脏停搏，心脏骤停
computed tomography	计算机断层扫描术
oxygen bottle	氧气瓶
intravenous (IV) pole	输液架，静脉输液架
life-critical	adj. 生命攸关的
homogeneous [ˌhəʊməˈdʒiːniəs]	adj. 同种类的，均质的
cardiologist [ˌkɑːdiˈɒlədʒɪst]	n. 心脏病医生，心脏病学家
over-the-counter	adj. 无需处方可买到的，非处方的
mammography [mæˈmɒgrəfi]	n. 乳房 X 射线照相术
wheelchair [ˈwiːltʃeə]	n. 轮椅
nebulizer [ˈnebjəlaɪzə]	n. 雾化器

physical disability	残疾，肢体残疾
insulin pump	胰岛素泵
paramedic [ˌpærə'medɪk]	n. 急救医士
de facto [ˌdeɪ 'fæktəʊ]	adj. 实际上存在的（不一定合法）

Key Sentences

1. Human factors engineering (HFE) is the application of knowledge about human capabilities (physical, sensory, emotional, and intellectual) and limitations to the design and development of tools, devices, systems, environments, and organizations. HFE might also be called human factors, ergonomics, human engineering, usability engineering, or human-computer interaction (HCI).

参考译文：人因工程是研究人的能力（身体、感官、情感和思维）和局限性，并将其应用于工具、设备、系统、环境和组织的设计和开发的一门学科。人因工程也称为人因学、人机工效学、人体工程学、可用性工程学或人机交互。

2. Usability testing is arguably the cornerstone of the human factors engineering process. It is good business to thoroughly evaluate a device's user interface before commercial deployment, when use error can put patients and users at risk.

参考译文：可用性测试可以说是人因工程的基石。在产品上市之前彻底评估医疗器械的用户界面是很有意义的，因为使用错误会使患者和用户面临风险。

3. The term "accessibility" has traditionally been associated with architectural features, such as sidewalks, building entrances, and restrooms. Features such as curb cuts, automatic doors, and restroom stalls equipped with assist bars are products of regulations and political activism that have improved accessibility to public spaces.

参考译文：在传统意义上来说，术语"可达性"与一些建筑特点相关，如人行道、建筑入口和卫生间。例如，便于轮椅通行的斜坡道、自动门，以及配有扶手的卫生间隔板门等都是有关法规和政策的产物，它们改善了公共空间的可达性。

Further Readings

Optimize User Interactions to Enhance Safety and Effectiveness

Make Devices Error-Tolerant and Fail in a Safe Manner

Consistent with modern principles of resilience engineering, device designs should be tolerant of error to minimize harm to users or patients. Design approaches to enhance error tolerance include designing for the device to fail safely, considering the overall context of use, providing more information about the implications of use actions, making use errors or unwanted deviations visible to users, making potential risks more visible to users, and facilitating error recovery.

A basic engineering design principle is to fail safely. For example, a household iron shuts itself off if the user fails to do so. Failing in a safe manner is even more important for medical devices because patient lives are at stake. The concept of failing in a safe manner can be extended from electromechanical failures to use errors. For example, a laser treatment device should not fire if the emergency stop control is inoperative. Moreover, if a critical device component like a control fails, an alternative means of control should be provided. For example, if a pump's stop switch is damaged, a mechanical means of ceasing pump action should be readily apparent to the user.

Avoid Physical Strain, Repetitive Motions, and Cumulative Traumas

The repetitious nature of many medical procedures, such as firmly squeezing and releasing a surgical stapler, puts users at risk of repetitive motion or cumulative trauma disorders. Designers should try to reduce the number of repetitive actions required to operate a device. They should also try to minimize manually applied forces, eliminate pressure points between devices and users, and allow users to maintain neutral joint positions. Designs should limit the amount of time users are required to apply a constant force (e.g. continuously squeeze the handles on a grasping tool), even if the force is relatively small. A relatively simple design change will often achieve these goals.

Help Users Anticipate Future Events

To provide the best patient care, clinicians generally try to predict the most likely course of disease manifestations and therapeutic interventions. In other words, users try to figure out what is going to happen rather than simply what is currently happening or what happened in the past. This is especially true for situations in which a user is delivering a therapy that can have a dramatic effect on the patient's physiological state, such as the intravenous delivery of a blood pressure medication. When possible, designs should help users "see ahead". For example, a monitoring device might model or forecast patient variables in the next 5, 10, and 30 minutes. A gas insufflation device might provide an indication of when a desired pressure (or volume) within the body cavity will be attained.

Confirm Important Actions

Confirmation messages can serve an important or even critical purpose, considering that some user actions are irreversible and could lead to injury. Therefore, even though some users might regard confirmation messages as a wasted extra step, the benefit of such messages in safety-critical situations often outweighs the annoyance they cause. The benefits of confirmation messages should be substantiated through user testing to ensure that they do not replace one problem with another, such as users confirming their actions without thinking about it (i.e. performing tasks in a rote manner).

Make Critical Controls Robust and Guard Them

Medical devices might be handled roughly, particularly if used outdoors or under emergency conditions (e.g. patient resuscitation procedures or "codes"). Because all medical devices might be dropped or bumped, all user interfaces need to be designed to prevent accidental actuation of critical controls. For example, incidental contact with a device's front panel should not deactivate a device or alter a critical control setting. Many medical devices have physically guarded power buttons and require users to confirm critical adjustments.

Clarify Operational Modes

One way that designers seek to simplify medical device is to incorporate multiple operational modes. In principle, multiple operational modes are a sensible way to facilitate tasks and to limit user exposure to extraneous capabilities. However, problems can arise if the user does not realize the medical device is in the wrong mode (often called "mode error"). For example, critical care nurse was observed inadvertently monitoring patients using a monitor that was in Demo mode and thus was not accurately portraying the patients' actual physiological conditions. Although Demo mode might be a useful feature for sales personnel or during user training, inadvertent conversion by a clinician to this mode during actual patient care is a life-threatening situation and puts the manufacturer at tremendous liability and market reputation risks. Accordingly, designers should make operational modes and their characteristics readily apparent.

Employ Redundant Coding

Redundant coding of displays and controls can be a powerful way to ensure reliable device operation. The concern is that a user, who could be fatigued and distracted, might actuate the wrong control or mistake one value for another (e.g. a "1" for a "7"). These kinds of use errors are less likely if displays and controls employ more than one means of coding. Coding options include varying the size, shape, color, texture, markings, or placement of the user-interface element. For example, anesthesia machines use redundant coding (knob color, shape, texture, and position) to ensure that users turn the correct knob to increase the flow of 100% oxygen versus air or nitrous oxide.

Design to Prevent User Confusion

While trying to make devices compatible, designers should also consider when it is appropriate to make devices or device components distinct. For example, it is advantageous to distinguish power cable receptacles from sensor cable receptacles, thereby avoiding circumstances in which a user might plug a patient sensor lead into an AC outlet and shock the patient. Devices and their components can be distinguished using the coding methods. In the case of plugs and receptacles, size and shape coding are particularly appropriate, making it impossible for a user to fit a particular plug into the wrong receptacle.

Do Not Neglect Device Appeal

Human factors are not only about safe and effective task performance, but also about user satisfaction. Designers should try to make medical devices pleasing to use. One payoff from making devices visually appealing is that patients, particularly children, might find them less frightening. Moreover, users might be more motivated to use appealing devices properly. Added appeal might also increase vigilance and job satisfaction. For example, a user might pay closer attention to a display with a pleasing appearance that also draws attention to important information than to one that has a garish appearance. A user might be drawn to a portable patient monitor because of design qualities that extend beyond functionality to boost appeal (e.g. an enclosure that looks attractive and easy to handle). The same can be said of tools that look comfortable to hold. However, medical devices intended for use in the home should not look like toys or children might try to play with them.

Part III   About Submitting a Paper

Unit 13   Considering About Preparing a Paper

Academic writing, especially a paper, has always played a large and central role for students all over the world.

It teaches students to analyze. A good paper usually requires students to look at somebody else's work or ideas and then form an informed opinion on it. Instead of merely describing the work of other people, students have to think about why it has been carried out and which uses its findings may have for the future. This type of writing makes students take in what they have read and decide how much importance it holds for their subject.

It allows students to convey their understanding. When students learn about a complex subject at university, it can be difficult for them to explain what they have understood if they struggle with academic writing. Papers give students the chance to explain what they have learnt by using the correct terminology and styles to make the information understood by others.

13.1   Types of Papers

The following types of manuscript may be submitted for consideration.

● Review—Potential notable author is actively encouraged to contact the Editor-in-Chief with a short summary of his/her proposed topic.

● Research paper—It describes original work. The kind of research may vary depending on the topic (experiments, survey, interview, questionnaire, etc.), but authors need to collect and analyze raw data and conduct an original study. The research paper will be based on the analysis and interpretation of the data collected.

● Short communication—It reports important observations that are usually preliminary in nature. It is suitable for the presentation of research that extends previously published research, including the reporting of additional controls and confirmatory results in other settings, as well as negative results.

- Technical note — It should normally describe a technical development, could be a software package for example. It is a short article giving a brief description of a specific development, technique or procedure, or it may describe a modification of an existing technique, procedure or device.

13.2　Choice to Publish Open Access

You can either choose to publish gold open access or make your article available via green open access options.

Gold open access means that the final published version of your article (or version of record) is permanently and freely available online for anyone, anywhere to read. An article publishing charge (APC) is usually applicable if you publish gold open access.

Green open access, also known as self-archiving, is when you post an earlier version of your manuscript in repositories and online. This enables you to share your article without having to pay an APC.

13.3　Use of Inclusive Language

Inclusive language acknowledges diversity, conveys respect to all people, is sensitive to differences, and promotes equal opportunities. Articles should make no assumptions about the beliefs or commitments of any reader, should contain nothing which might imply that one individual is superior to another on the grounds of race, sex, culture or any other characteristic, and should use inclusive language throughout. Authors should ensure that writing is free from bias, for instance by using "he or she", "his/her" instead of "he" or "his", and by making use of job titles that are free of stereotyping (e.g. "chairperson" instead of "chairman" and "flight attendant" instead of "stewardess").

13.4　Article Structure

There are many types of articles. The article structure for the content will vary depending on the topic. Regardless of the article you write, there is a basic structure you should follow to be effective.

Subdivision—Numbered Sections

Divide your article into clearly defined and numbered sections. Subsections should be numbered 1.1 (then 1.1.1, 1.1.2, ...), 1.2, etc. (the abstract is not included in section numbering). Use this numbering also for internal cross-referencing: do not just refer to "the text". Any subsection may be given a brief heading. Each heading should appear on its own separate line.

Introduction

State the objectives of the work and provide an adequate background, avoiding a detailed literature survey or a summary of the results.

Material and Methods

Provide sufficient details to allow the work to be reproduced by an independent researcher. Methods that are already published should be summarized, and indicated by a reference. If quoting directly from a previously published method, use quotation marks and also cite the source. Any modifications to existing methods should also be described.

Theory/Calculation

A *Theory* section should extend, not repeat, the background to the article already dealt with in the *Introduction* and lay the foundation for further work. In contrast, a *Calculation* section represents a practical development from a theoretical basis.

Results

Results should be clear and concise.

Discussion

This should explore the significance of the results of the work, not repeat them. A combined *Results and Discussion* section is often appropriate. Avoid extensive citations and discussion of published literature.

Conclusions

The main conclusions of the study may be presented in a short *Conclusions* section, which may stand alone or form a subsection of a *Discussion* or *Results and Discussion* section.

Appendices

If there is more than one appendix, they should be identified as A, B, etc. Formulae and equations in appendices should be given separate numbering: Eq. (A.1), Eq. (A.2), etc.; in a subsequent appendix, Eq. (B.1) and so on. Similarly for tables and figures: Table A.1; Fig. A.1, etc.

13.5   Role of the Funding Source

It is requested to identify who provided financial support for the conduct of the research and/or preparation of the article and to briefly describe the role of the sponsor(s), if any, in study design; in the collection, analysis and interpretation of data; in the writing of the report;

and in the decision to submit the article for publication. If the funding source(s) had no such involvement then this should be stated.

13.6 Declaration of Interest

All authors must disclose any financial and personal relationships with other people or organizations that could inappropriately influence (bias) their work. Examples of potential competing interests include employment, consultancies, stock ownership, honoraria, paid expert testimony, patent applications/registrations, and grants or other funding. Authors must disclose any interests in two places. (1) A summary declaration of interest statement in the title page file (if double-blind) or the manuscript file (if single-blind). If there are no interests to declare then please state "Declarations of interest: none". This summary statement will be ultimately published if the article is accepted. (2) Detailed disclosures as part of a separate Declaration of Interest form, which forms part of the journal's official records. It is important for potential interests to be declared in both places and that the information matches.

13.7 Peer Review

All contributions will be initially assessed by the editor for suitability for the journal. Papers deemed suitable are then typically sent to a minimum of two independent expert reviewers to assess the scientific quality of the paper. The editor is responsible for the final decision regarding acceptance or rejection of articles.

13.8 General Steps to Prepare a Journal Paper

To prepare a journal article for publication, the following steps are helpful.

1. Pick a Journal

Deciding where to submit your work can be difficult, especially with a number of academic journals available. Key factors to consider are listed below.

- How well your research fits with the focus of the journal (try looking for a specialist journal that covers the subject of your paper).
- The accessibility of the journal, including which databases it is listed on.
- Whether the journal is available in print, online or both.
- How often it publishes per year and the time the review process takes.
- The impact and status of the journal.

Do a little research on the journals available in your subject area and see which ones carry articles most like your own. And remember that you should only submit to one journal at a time.

2. Read the Submission Guidelines

Once you have decided on a journal, check the publisher's website for submission guidelines. These will usually be named something like "Author Instructions" or "Submission Procedures".

These documents provide advice on a number of things regarding how to prepare a journal article for publication, including:

(1) how a paper should be written (e.g. punctuation preferences);

(2) how a paper should be formatted prior to submission;

(3) which referencing style to use and how to list sources;

(4) how to submit your paper and any extra documentation required (e.g. whether you need an abstract and key words to go with your paper).

Following these guidelines is crucial, so check the instructions carefully.

3. Editing and Proofreading

Use the editing process to make sure your article fits your chosen journal. To do this, check the submission guidelines and what the journal usually publishes before you begin redrafting. You may not need to make major changes, but this could still affect how you frame your arguments.

We also suggest having a professional editor or proofreader check your writing before submitting. This will ensure that your paper is error free and as easy to read as possible. And if you do hire a professional, make sure to let them know whether the publisher has a style guide available.

4. First Impressions — The Title and Cover Letter

Making a good first impression will not hurt your chances of getting published. One way to do this is by picking a great title for your article. Some factors should be considered.

- Ideally, it should indicate exactly what you were investigating.
- Use a subtitle to provide extra information if required.
- Try to be clear and concise (aim for a maximum of 12 words in a title).
- Avoid undefined initialisms and acronyms.
- Puns or humor in a title can be fun, but keep in mind that they could be inappropriate or confusing for international readers who may not speak English as a first language.

You will also need to prepare a cover letter before submitting your work. This should briefly summarize your research, but do not go into too much detail. Instead, focus on providing context for your research, e.g. your academic history and interests and what your work contributes to the subject area.

5. Revise and Resubmit

Whenever you submit an article to a journal, you will receive feedback from reviewers. This may be part of a rejection, but you will usually need to make changes even if the journal accepts your paper.

Whatever the result, do not let critical feedback get you down. Even if it seems harsh, you can learn from it and use it to make revisions before you resubmit the paper (or submit it elsewhere).

13.9　Online Submission

Authors are free to submit their manuscripts electronically by online submission system. Editor-in-chief will return the manuscript(s) that do not follow the requirements or that are otherwise deemed unsuitable for publication to the author(s) for revision. Authors are responsible for the mistakes made in details, such as the author names, institutional affiliations, etc.

13.10　Publication Policy

Submitted article for publication must not be previously published, or sent to another journal for publication. The manuscript should contain nothing that is abusive, defamatory, libelous, fraudulent, or illegal. Articles should be either theoretical or research-based articles.

13.11　Plagiarism Policy

Articles submitted are supposed to be original. Plagiarism of other published articles, without appropriate attribution, is unethical. If the editors or reviewers suspect plagiarism, submitted articles will be checked with plagiarism detection software. In the case of a submitted article having been found to have been totally or substantially published elsewhere, the submitted article is rejected outright. The editors may ban the authors from submitting to the journal for a defined time period. The author attests the following declaration.

(1) None of the part of manuscript is plagiarized from other sources.

(2) Proper reference is provided for all contents extracted from other sources.

(3) Strong action will be taken against cases of plagiarism.

Words and Expressions

academic writing	学术性写作
terminology [ˌtɜːmɪˈnɒlədʒi]	n.（某学科的）术语
research paper	研究论文
short communication	短讯，研究简报
technical note	技术说明，技术注解
gold open access	金色开放获取
green open access	绿色开放获取
article publishing charge (APC)	文章出版费
manuscript [ˈmænjʊskrɪpt]	n. 手稿
inclusive language	包容性语言
theoretical basis	理论基础
declaration of interest	利益声明
double-blind	双盲
single-blind	单盲
author instruction	作者说明，作者指南
submission procedure	投稿步骤
cover letter	投稿信

Key Sentences

1. It teaches students to analyze. A good paper usually requires students to look at somebody else's work or ideas and then form an informed opinion on it. Instead of merely describing the work of other people, students have to think about why it has been carried out and which uses its findings may have for the future. This type of writing makes students take in what they have read and decide how much importance it holds for their subject.

参考译文：（论文写作）教会学生如何分析。撰写一篇好的论文通常需要学生阅读别人的著作或观点，并在此基础上形成自己的论点。学生们不仅要描述前人的研究，还必须思考为什么要进行这项研究，以及研究结果对未来可能会有什么影响。这种类型的写作让学生了解他们所读的内容，从而决定该研究对他们自己的课题的重要性如何。

2. It allows students to convey their understanding. When students learn about a complex subject at university, it can be difficult for them to explain what they have understood if they struggle with academic writing. Papers give students the chance to explain

what they have learnt by using the correct terminology and styles to make the information understood by others.

参考译文：（论文写作）让学生表达其观点成为可能。当学生在大学里学习一门复杂的学科时，如果他们在学术性写作方面有困难，就很难解释清楚他们所理解的内容。论文让学生有机会通过使用正确的术语和文体来解释他们所学的内容，从而使其他人理解这些信息。

Further Readings

Science Citation Index and Science Citation Index Expanded

Science Citation Index (SCI) and Engineering Index (EI), two world famous major science and technology literature retrieval systems, are internationally recognized as the scientific statistics and scientific evaluation of the main retrieval tools, among them with SCI being the most important.

SCI was founded by the American Institute for Scientific Information (ISI) in 1961, and it is the publication of the citation database covering life science, clinical medicine, physical chemistry, agriculture, biology, veterinary medicine, engineering and technical aspects of integrated retrieval periodicals, especially reflecting the academic level of science research. Its citation index shows a unique scientific reference value, and occupies an important position in academia.

Web of Science (WoS) is an online subscription-based Scientific Citation Indexing (SCI) service originally produced by the Institute for Scientific Information (ISI). The Science Citation Index Expanded (SCIE) is the larger version of SCI which covers more than 8,500 notable and significant journals, across 150 disciplines, from 1900 to the present. SCIE is similar to the SCI except for the two differences.

(1) Impact factor. SCI has non-zero impact factor but SCIE journals are just ranked for impact factor.

(2) Storage format. Both SCI and SCIE are available online. However, SCI is available on CD/DVD format but SCIE is not.

Engineering Index

Engineering Village is an essential resource for students, researchers and faculty to stay up-to-date in their field, acquire knowledge in new areas, set up research proposals and write papers. It is the leading information discovery platform specifically designed by and for the engineering community.

Engineering Index (EI) is the broadest and most complete engineering literature database available in the world. It provides a truly holistic and global view of peer reviewed and indexed publications with over 20 million records from 77 countries across 190 engineering disciplines. Every record is carefully selected and indexed using the Engineering Index Thesaurus to ensure discovery and retrieval of engineering-specific literature that engineering students and professionals can rely on. By using EI, engineers can be confident that information is relevant, complete, accurate and of high quality.

Here are the EI related areas.

- Applied Physics, including Optics;
- Bioengineering and Biotechnology;
- Food Science and Technology;
- Materials Science;
- Instrumentation, including Medical Devices;
- Nanotechnology.

附录 A　主要学术机构

1. International Federation for Medical and Biological Engineering (IFMBE)

The International Federation for Medical and Biological Engineering (IFMBE), founded in 1959, is a nonprofit scientific organization of independent affiliates in 30 countries. IFMBE members include biomedical engineers, technologists and technicians, clinical engineers, rehabilitation engineers, physicians, medical physicists, and biologists. The objectives of the IFMBE are to generate and disseminate information to the international biomedical engineering community, provide a forum, encourage research and application of biomedical engineering knowledge in support of life quality and cost-effective health care, stimulate international cooperation in the field, and encourage educational programs in biomedical engineering.

IFMBE publishes the monthly journal of *Medical & Biological Engineering & Computing*, the bimonthly news reports The IFMBE News, and the annual IFMBE Directory of affiliates and committees. In collaboration with the International Organization for Medical Physics, IFMBE organizes a world conference every three years.

The IFMBE Joint Working Group on the Implications and Assessment of Biomedical Innovations seeks to convene engineers and medical scientists to explore social and economic influences of biomedical innovations, develop and apply assessment methods, and analyze means by which social and economic factors should influence engineering decisions.

IFMBE consults with the International Electric Commission and the International Measurement Confederation in developing standards, e.g. for digital imaging. IFMBE affiliates participate on technology assessment councils, standards and safety boards, and other efforts related to international standards in medical device safety.

2. American Institute for Medical and Biological Engineering (AIMBE)

The American Institute for Medical and Biological Engineering (AIMBE) is a non-profit organization headquartered in Washington, D.C., representing the most accomplished individuals in the fields of medical and biological engineering. No other organization can bring together academia, industry, government, and scientific societies to form a highly influential community advancing medical and biological engineering. AIMBE's mission is to provide leadership and advocacy in medical and biological engineering for the benefit of society.

AIMBE is the authoritative voice and advocate for the value of medical and biological engineering to society. It is an organization of leaders in medical and biological engineering, consisting of academic, industrial, professional societies, and elected fellows. Its main responsibilities are listed below.

- Communicate objectively with the U.S. and state government agencies, Congress, industry, academia, and professional societies by advocating and providing service to the public via medical and biological engineering.

- Contribute to public policy advancing medical and biological engineering for benefit society.

- Work to ensure appropriate private and public investment to advance medical and biological engineering translational research and innovation.

- Inspire, educate, and involve young people who will be the future leaders of medical and biological engineering.

- Promote intersociety and multi-disciplinary cooperation within the medical and biological engineering community.

- Recognize and honor achievements and contributions to the field of medical and biological engineering.

3. IEEE Engineering in Medicine and Biology Society (EMBS)

Helping to facilitate and accelerate the advancement of engineering in healthcare is IEEE's Engineering in Medicine and Biology Society. IEEE is the largest professional society in the world, with nearly 400,000 members worldwide. As one of IEEE's 38 societies, IEEE EMBS is the largest professional society dedicated to the technology of biomedicine. EMBS is the society that is improving and advancing technology for better diagnosis and treatment of chronic and acute healthcare maladies.

The work of biomedical engineers touches so many fields and specialties. And many areas of research overlap and borrow from one another. So, it is important to have an organization like IEEE EMBS that brings together professionals focusing on various disciplines to advance science and medicine at a faster pace than would otherwise be possible if everyone worked in silos.

Whether you develop or use medical technology, IEEE EMBS provides a common link to the science behind healthcare technology. Our members hail from industry, academic institutions, hospitals, labs and government agencies. Every year, at the Annual EMBS Conference, members exchange practical ideas in forums dedicated to medical product development.

While EMBS members are working in different areas of the very broad field of biomedical engineering, we share a common goal of better understanding biology and medical systems to ultimately improve global health and enhance quality of life.

Membership in IEEE EMBS provides a forum for other, like-minded individuals to exchange ideas and help advance research more rapidly. Members are given access to comprehensive coverage and breaking news on emerging trends, mature and cutting-edge technologies and research breakthroughs.

4. Biomedical Engineering Society (BMES)

The Biomedical Engineering Society (BMES) is the professional society for biomedical engineering and bioengineering. Founded in early 1968, the society now boasts over 5,000 members and is growing rapidly.

BMES serves as the lead society and professional home for biomedical engineering and bioengineering. Its leadership in accreditation, potential licensure, publications, scientific meetings, global programs, and diversity initiatives, as well as its commitment to ethics, all serve its mission to promote and enhance knowledge and education in biomedical engineering and bioengineering worldwide and its utilization for human health and well-being.

5. The Chinese Society of Biomedical Engineering (CSBME)

Founded in 1980, the Chinese Society of Biomedical Engineering (CSBME) is a national first-class society, which is rated 4A by the Ministry of Civil Affairs. It is one of the professional societies in China that integrates scientific research, teaching, clinical practice and research and development.

At present, CSBME has 34 branches (professional committees) and 17 working committees. Among the 23,000 members of the society, there are senior, middle-aged and young professionals in the field of biomedical engineering, including academicians of the Chinese Academy of Sciences and the Chinese Academy of Engineering, Changjiang Scholars, distinguished professors, clinical medicine experts, experts and entrepreneurs in the development and production of medical devices.

Biomedical engineering uses engineering science and technology to promote the progress of biological and medical sciences. It is one of the fastest growing disciplines in the world. Since its establishment for 40 years, CSBME has been fully leading the progress of biomedical engineering in China in terms of discipline construction and promoting the combination of production, learning, research and medicine. Through the organization of academic exchanges at home and abroad, CSBME edits and publishes professional books and periodicals, carries out popular science activities, and disseminates scientific spirit and ideas. CSBME organizes members and scientific and technological workers to provide suggestions for the development of science and technology, and to participate in the investigation, approval and evaluation organized by State Council, the National Development and Reform Commission, the Ministry of Science and Technology, the Ministry of Industry and Information Technology, the National Health Commission, the National Medical Products Administration, the National Natural Science Foundation of China, the Chinese Academy of Engineering, etc. The transfer of government functions promotes the development of science and technology.

The academic journals sponsored by CSBME include *Chinese Journal of Biomedical Engineering*, *Chinese Journal of Biomedical Engineering* (English Edition), *Chinese Journal of Cardiac Pacing and Electrophysiology* and *Chinese Journal of Hemorheology*. Among them, *Chinese Journal of Biomedical Engineering* has long been included in China Science Citation Database (CSCD), Chinese Core Journals of Peking University and Chinese Core Journals of science and Technology (CJCR), and the impact factors of CJCR have always been in the forefront of this field.

In the future, CSBME will focus on the three themes of "Strengthening Ability, Increasing Connotation and Building Mechanism" to establish a brand, build a professional think tank, improve the innovation mechanism, strengthen the cultural construction, lead the development direction of the discipline, enhance the ability of international exchange and cooperation, and build a first-class science and technology association with important international influence.

附录 B 常用英文期刊列表

Table B.1

英文期刊名称	英文期刊名称
Acta Biomaterialia	Biomedical Microdevices
Acta of Bioengineering and Biomechanics	Biomedical Signal Processing and Control
Acta Pharmaceutica Sinica B	Biopreservation and Biobanking
Acta Physiologiae Plantarum	Biosensors & Bioelectronics
Advanced Drug Delivery Reviews	Biotechnology & Biotechnological Equipment
Advances in Mechanical Engineering	Biotechnology and Genetic Engineering Reviews
Analytica Chimica Acta	British Dental Journal
Analytical and Bioanalytical Chemistry	Carbohydrate Polymers
Annals of Biomedical Engineering	Cardiovascular Engineering
Annals of Microbiology	Cell and Tissue Banking
Annual Review of Biomedical Engineering	Chemical Journal of Chinese Universities (Chinese)
Annual Review of Biomedical Engineering Biomaterials	Chemical Speciation & Bioavailability
AoB Plants	Chemistry Letters
Applied and Environmental Microbiology	Chinese Journal of Analytical Chemistry
Applied Biological Chemistry	Clinical Oral Implants Research
Applied Thermal Engineering	Clinical Biomechanics
Artificial Cells, Blood Substitutes, and Immobilization Biotechnology	Coatings
Artificial Intelligence in Medicine	Colloid Journal
Artificial Organs	Computer Methods in Biomechanics and Biomedical Engineering
Australasian Physical & Engineering Sciences in Medicine	Computers and Electronics in Agriculture
Biofabrication	Computers in Biology and Medicine
Biomaterials	Critical Reviews in Biotechnology
Biomechanics and Modeling in Mechanobiology	Cryoletters
BioMed Research International	Current Microbiology
BioMedical Engineering Online	Dialysis & Transplantation
Biomedical Engineering/Biomedizinische Technik	Drying Technology
Bio-Medical Materials and Engineering	Ecological Research

英文期刊名称	英文期刊名称
Electronic Journal of Biotechnology	Journal of Biotechnology
European Neuropsychopharmacology	Journal of Buon
Expert Review of Medical Devices	Journal of Dairy Science
FEMS Microbiology Letters	Journal of Genetics and Genomics
Flora	Journal of Healthcare Engineering
Free Radical Biology & Medicine	Journal of Magnetic Resonance
Frontiers in Aging Neuroscience	Journal of Mechanics in Medicine and Biology
Frontiers in Genetics	Journal of Medical and Biological Engineering
Frontiers in Microbiology	Journal of Medical Devices
IEEE Engineering in Medicine and Biology Magazine	Journal of Medical Devices—Transactions of the ASME
IEEE Transactions on Biomedical Engineering	Journal of Medical Imaging and Health Informatics
IEEE Transactions on Neural Systems and Rehabilitation Engineering	Journal of Nanobiotechnology
IEEE Transactions on Biomedical Circuits and Systems	Journal of Neural Engineering
IEEE Transactions on Medical Imaging	Journal of NeuroEngineering and Rehabilitation
Immunology Letters	Journal of the American Heart Association
Interdisciplinary Sciences: Computational Life Sciences	Journal of the Mechanical Behavior of Biomedical Materials
International Journal for Numerical Methods in Biomedical Engineering	Journal of Tissue Engineering
International Journal of Aerospace Engineering	Journal of Tissue Engineering and Regenerative Medicine
International Journal of Biological Macromolecules	Journal of X-Ray Science and Technology
International Journal of Clinical and Experimental Medicine	Lasers in Medical Science
International Journal of Computer Assisted Radiology and Surgery	Letters in Applied Microbiology
International Journal of Heat and Mass Transfer	Materials
Journal of Alloys and Compounds	Medical & Biological Engineering & Computing
Journal of Applied Biomaterials & Biomechanics	Medical Engineering & Physics
Journal of Applied Biomechanics	Medical Image Analysis
Journal of Applied Spectroscopy	Medical Physics
Journal of Biomaterials Applications	Microbial Pathogenesis
Journal of Biomaterials Science	Microchimica ACTA
Journal of Biomechanics	Minimally Invasive Therapy & Allied Technologies
Journal of Biomedical Engineering	Molecular Simulation
Journal of Biomedical Materials Research—Part B: Applied Biomaterials	Molecules
Journal of Biomedical Materials Research—Part A	Nanomedicine

续表

英文期刊名称	英文期刊名称
Optics and Lasers in Engineering	Progress in Biochemistry and Biophysics
Optik	Redox Report
Organogenesis	Regenerative Medicine
Perspectives in Plant Ecology, Evolution and Systematics	Research on Chemical Intermediates
Physica Medica: European Journal of Medical Physics	Scientific Reports
Physical Review Letters	Sensors and Actuators B: Chemical
Physics in Medicine & Biology	Shock and Vibration
Physiological Measurement	Spectroscopy and Spectral Analysis
Phytochemistry	Sports Biomechanics
Plant Biology	Surface Review and Letters
Plant Disease	Talanta
Plant Ecology	Technology and Health Care
PLOS ONE	The International Journal of Artificial Organs
Polymers for Advanced Technologies	Trends in Biotechnology
Postharvest Biology and Technology	Ultrasonic Imaging
Process Biochemistry	World Journal of Gastroenterology

附录 C　常用中文期刊列表

Table C.1

中文期刊名称	中文期刊名称
《中国生物医学工程学报》	《生殖医学杂志》
《生物医学工程学杂志》	《现代仪器与医疗》
《医用生物力学》	《影像科学与光化学》
《中国医学物理学杂志》	《中国介入影像与治疗学》
《北京生物医学工程》	《中国临床医学影像杂志》
《生物安全学报》	《中国医学工程》
《生物骨科材料与临床研究》	《中国医学影像技术》
《生物技术》	《中国医学影像学杂志》
《生物技术通报》	《中华超声影像学杂志》
《生物技术通讯》	《中华生物医学工程杂志》
《生物学杂志》	《中华物理医学与康复杂志》
《生物医学工程学进展》	《中国心脏起搏与心电生理杂志》
《生物医学工程研究》	《中国血液流变学杂志》
《生物医学工程与临床》	《国际生物医学工程杂志》

附录 D　词汇表

A

academic writing	学术性写作
accelerometer [ək͵selə'rɒmɪtə]	n. 加速度计
acid-base balance	酸碱平衡
active medical device	有源医疗器械
adhesive dressings	胶粘敷料
agriculture ['ægrɪ͵kʌltʃə]	n. 农业
ailment ['eɪlmənt]	n. 小病，轻病
algorithm ['ælgərɪðəm]	n. 算法
alternating current	交流
Alzheimer's disease	阿尔茨海默病
amputation [͵æmpjə'teɪʃən]	n. 截肢
amputee [͵æmpjə'ti:]	n. 被截肢者
analogue to digital conversion (ADC)	模数转换
analyte ['ænəlaɪt]	n.（被）分析物，分解物
anatomy [ə'nætəmi]	n. 解剖
anesthesia and respiratory devices	麻醉和呼吸器械
anesthesia disposables	麻醉一次性用品
anesthesia machine	麻醉机
ankle brachial index	踝臂指数
anthropometry [͵ænθrə'pɒmɪtrɪ]	n. 人体测量，人体测量学
antibody ['æntɪ͵bɒdi]	n. 抗体
antigen ['æntɪdʒən]	n. 抗原（能激发人体产生抗体）
aperture ['æpətʃə]	n. 小孔
archaeologic [͵ɑ:kɪə'lɒdʒɪk]	adj. 考古学的，考古学上的
arrhythmia [ə'rɪðmɪə]	n. 心律不齐（失常）
article publishing charge (APC)	文章出版费
artificial heart	人工心脏
artificial limb	假肢
artificial organ	人工器官
atrophic [æ'trɒfɪk]	adj. 萎缩的

author instruction	作者说明，作者指南
axial ['æksiəl]	*adj.* 横断的，轴线的

B

bandage ['bændɪdʒ]	*n.* 绷带
bandpass filter	带通滤光片
basophil ['beɪsəfɪl]	*n.* 嗜碱性粒细胞
bedpan ['bedpæn]	*n.*（卧床患者用的）便盆
benign prostatic hyperplasia (BPH) treatment	良性前列腺增生的治疗
biconcave [baɪ'kɒnkeɪv]	*adj.* 双凹面的，两面凹的
bilirubin [ˌbɪlɪ'ruːbɪn]	*n.* 胆红素
biocompatible [ˌbaɪəʊkəm'pætɪbl]	*adj.* 生物相容的
bioinformatics [ˌbaɪəʊɪnfə'mætɪks]	*n.* 生物信息学
bioinstrumentation [baɪəʊˌɪnstrʊmen'teɪʃn]	*n.* 生物仪器
biomaterial ['baɪəʊməˌtɪəriəl]	*n.* 生物材料，生物材料学
biomechanics [ˌbaɪəʊmə'kænɪks]	*n.* 生物力学
biomechatronics [baɪəʊˌmekə'trɒnɪks]	*n.* 生物机械电子学
biomedical engineering (BME)	生物医学工程
biomedical instrumentation	生物医学仪器
biomedical sensor	生物医学传感器
biopsy ['baɪɒpsi]	*n.* 活体标本检查
blocking bar	阻塞棒
blood biomarker	血液生物标志物
blood glucose meter	血糖计
blood glucose test strip	血糖试纸
blood perfusion	血液灌注
bone morphing	骨变形

C

cannula ['kænjʊlə]	*n.*（输药等的）套管，插管
capstone project	顶点课程，高级论文或高级研讨会
carbon dioxide	二氧化碳
cardiac arrest	心脏停搏，心脏骤停
cardiac assist	心脏辅助
cardiac or respiration phase	心脏或呼吸周期
cardiac rhythm management (CRM)	心脏节律管理
cardiologist [ˌkɑːdi'ɒlədʒɪst]	*n.* 心脏病医生，心脏病学家
cardiovascular biomechanics	心血管生物力学

cardiovascular surgery	心血管外科
cataract surgery	白内障手术
catheter ['kæθɪtə]	n. 导管（如导尿管）
cathode ray oscilloscope (CRO)	阴极射线示波器
cell counting	细胞计数
cell diffusion	细胞扩散
cerebrospinal fluid	脑脊液
cerebrospinal fluid pressure	脑脊液压力
chart recorder	图表记录仪，图表记录器
chronic venous leg ulcer	慢性下肢静脉性溃疡
clinical engineering	临床工程
clinical thermometer	临床用体温计
coagulation [kəʊˌægjə'leɪʃn]	n. 凝固作用，凝结
cochlear implant	人工耳蜗
cognition [kɒg'nɪʃən]	n. 认知，感知，认识
cognitive function	认知功能
complementary [ˌkɒmplɪ'mentəri]	adj. 互补的，补充的
compression therapy	加压疗法
computed tomography	计算机断层扫描术
continuum mechanics	连续介质力学
contralateral [ˌkɒntrə'lætərəl]	adj. 对侧的
core body temperature	体核温度，体温
corrective lenses	矫正眼镜，矫正镜片
cortical surface	皮质表面
covariate [ˌkʌ'veəriət]	n. 协变量
cover letter	投稿信
CT scan	CT 扫描
cybernetics [ˌsaɪbə'netɪks]	n. 控制论

D

dampen ['dæmpən]	vt. 减弱，抑制
de facto [ˌdeɪ 'fæktəʊ]	adj. 实际上存在的（不一定合法）
declaration of interest	利益声明
dedicated instruments	专用仪器
defibrillator [di:'fɪbrəleɪtə]	n. 除颤器
deformable model	变形模型
demographics [ˌdemə'græfɪks]	n. 人口统计学

dental implant	牙科植入体
dexterity [dek'sterəti]	*n.* 敏捷，灵活
dialysis [daɪˈæləsɪs]	*n.* 透析
dialysis machine	透析机
digital to analogue conversion (DAC)	数模转换
diluent ['dɪljʊənt]	*n.* 稀释液
direct current	直流
disarticulation [ˌdɪsɑːˌtɪkjəˈleɪʃən]	*n.* 关节脱落，关节切断术
discriminator [dɪsˈkrɪmɪneɪtə]	*n.* 甄别器
disposable gloves	一次性手套
DNA sequencing	DNA 测序
double-blind	双盲
drainage ['dreɪnɪdʒ]	*n.* 排水
dual-source and dual-energy CT	双源双能 CT
dynamics [daɪˈnæmɪks]	*n.* 动力学

E

ear/nose/throat (E.N.T.) devices	耳鼻喉器械，五官科器械
eccrine ['ekrin]	*adj.* 外分泌的
effective resistance	有效电阻
elastic bandage	弹性绷带
elastic stockings	弹力袜
electrical potential	电势（位）
electrical pulse	电脉冲
electrical resistance	电阻
electrical signal	电信号
electrocardiograph [ɪˌlektrəʊˈkɑːdiəɡrɑːf]	*n.* 心电图描记器
electrochemical [ɪˌlektrəʊˈkemɪkəl]	*adj.* 电化学的
electroencephalography [iˌlektrəʊɪnˈsefələɡrɑːfi] (EEG)	*n.* 脑电图
electrolyte [ɪˈlektrəlaɪt]	*n.* 电解液，电解质
electromyography [ɪˌlektrəʊmaɪˈɒɡrəfi]	*n.* 肌电图学，肌电图检查
electron microscopy	电子显微镜术，电子显微术
electrophysiology [ɪˌlektrəʊˌfɪziˈɒlədʒɪ]	*n.* 电生理学
energy state diagram	能级图
eosinophil [ˌiːəˈsɪnəfil]	*n.* 嗜酸性粒细胞
ergonomics [ˌɜːɡəˈnɒmɪks]	*n.* 工效学
erythrocyte [ɪˈrɪθrəʊsaɪt]	*n.* 红细胞

examination gloves	检查手套
expenditure [ɪk'spendɪtʃə]	*n.* 支出，开支，费用
extension [ɪk'stenʃən]	*n.* 伸展

F

facial prosthetics	面部修复术
fallibility [ˌfælə'bɪləti]	*n.* 易错性，不可靠性
femur ['fiːmə]	*n.* 股骨
flexion ['flekʃn]	*n.* 屈曲
flexion-extension	屈伸
flow cytometry	流式细胞术
fluidic system	液流系统
fluorescence [flɔː'resns]	*n.* 荧光
fluorescence intensity	荧光强度
fluorophore-labeled antibody	荧光标记抗体
fluoroscopy [flʊə'rɒskəpɪ]	*n.* 荧光学，荧光透视法
foodstuff ['fuːdstʌf]	*n.* 食物，食品
forceps ['fɔːsep]	*n.* 镊子
forward scatter (FSC)	前向散射
fracture stabilization	骨折固定
frontal ['frʌntl]	*adj.* 冠状的
functional recovering	功能恢复
functional tissue	功能尚存的组织

G

gait & posture analysis	步态与姿势分析
gait analysis	步态分析
galvanic skin response	皮肤电反应
gauze dressings	纱布敷料
genetic engineering	基因工程
genomics [dʒə'nəʊmɪks]	*n.* 基因组学
glucose uptake	葡萄糖摄取
gold open access	金色开放获取
granulocyte ['grænjʊləˌsaɪt]	*n.* 粒细胞，有粒白细胞
green fluorescence protein (GFP)	绿色荧光蛋白
green open access	绿色开放获取
gut flora	肠道菌群

H

handheld smartphone	手持智能手机
handheld surgical instrument	手持式手术器械
harness ['hɑ:nəs]	n. 悬吊，背带，保护带
health care	医疗保健，医疗卫生
heart-lung machine	心肺机
heartbeat ['hɑ:tbi:t]	n. 心跳，心搏
hematology [ˌhi:mə'tɒlədʒɪ]	n. 血液学
hemocyte ['hi:məsaɪt]	n. 血细胞
hemoglobin [ˌhi:mə'gləʊbɪn]	n. 血红蛋白
hemorrhage ['hemərɪdʒ]	出血，（尤指大量的）失血
heterogeneous population	异质群体
hip and knee joint implant	髋膝关节植入物
homeostasis [ˌhəʊmiəʊ'steɪsɪs]	n. 体内稳态，内环境稳定
homogeneous [ˌhəʊmə'dʒi:nɪəs]	adj. 同种类的，均质的
hormone ['hɔ:məʊn]	n. 激素，荷尔蒙
human-computer interaction	人机交互
human error	人为失误
human factors engineering	人机工程学，人因工程学
hydrodynamic focusing	液流聚焦

I

image modality	图像模式，图像形态
imaging agent	显像剂
immunochemistry [ˌɪmjunəʊ'kemɪstrɪ]	n. 免疫化学
immunohematology [ˌɪmjʊnəʊˌhi:mə'tɒlədʒɪ]	n. 免疫血液学
immunological [ˌɪmjunə'lɒdʒɪkəl]	adj. 免疫学的
immunophenotyping	免疫表型
implant ['ɪmplɑ:nt]	n. （植入人体中的）移植物，植入物
implantable sensor	可植入式传感器
inclusive language	包容性语言
individualized medicine	个体化医疗，个体化医学
inertia [ɪ'nɜ:ʃə]	n. 惯性
inertial sensor	惯性传感器
infection [ɪn'fekʃən]	n. 感染
informative [ɪn'fɔ:mətɪv]	adj. 提供有用信息的
infusion pump	输液泵

ingestible sensor	可吸收式传感器
injury biomechanics	损伤生物力学
insulin pen	胰岛素笔
insulin pump	胰岛素泵
intact upper limb	健侧上肢
interchangeable[ˌɪntə'tʃeɪndʒəbəl]	*adj.* 可交换的，可互换的
interdisciplinary [ˌɪntəˌdɪsə'plɪnəri]	*adj.* 多学科的，跨学科的
International Electrotechnical Commission	国际电工委员会
interrogation point	检测点
interventional cardiology	介入心脏病学
interventional neurology	介入神经学
intraoperative [ˌɪntrə'ɒpərətɪv]	*adj.* 术中的
intravenous (IV) pole	输液架，静脉输液架
intuitive [ɪn'tjuːətɪv]	*adj.* 直觉的
invitro diagnostics (IVD)	体外诊断

J

joint motion	关节活动

K

kinematics [ˌkɪnɪ'mætɪks]	*n.* 运动学

L

lab-on-a-chip device	芯片上实验室器械
lancing device	切割器械，采血笔
laser beam	激光束
lateral and medial malleoli	外踝和内踝
latex ['leɪteks]	*n.*（天然）胶乳
leukocyte ['ljuːkəsaɪt]	*n.* 白细胞
life-critical	*adj.* 生命攸关的
ligament complexes	韧带复合体
light path	光程
lightweight ['laɪtweɪt]	*adj.* 轻量的，薄型的
lobularity	*n.* 分叶状结构
location sensor	位置感应器，位置传感器
locomotion [ˌləʊkə'məʊʃən]	*n.* 运动，探索，行进
long-pass filter	长波通滤光片
lower extremity	下肢
lower limb	下肢

lymphocyte ['limfəsaɪt]　　　　　　　　　　n. 淋巴细胞

M

magnetic [mæg'netɪk]　　　　　　　　　　adj. 有磁性的，磁性的

magnetic field　　　　　　　　　　　　　　磁场

magnetic resonance imaging (MRI)　　　　磁共振成像

mammography [mæ'mɒgrəfi]　　　　　　　n. 乳房 X 射线照相术

manuscript ['mænjʊskrɪpt]　　　　　　　　n. 手稿

measurand ['meʒərənd]　　　　　　　　　　n. 被测量

mechanical axis　　　　　　　　　　　　　　力线

mechanical vibration　　　　　　　　　　　机械振动

mechanism analysis　　　　　　　　　　　机构分析

medical gloves　　　　　　　　　　　　　　医用手套

medical thermometer　　　　　　　　　　　医用温度计

megakaryocyte [megə'kærɪəʊsaɪt]　　　　　n. 巨核细胞

membrane ['membreɪn]　　　　　　　　　　n.（细胞）膜

metabolic [ˌmetə'bɒlɪk]　　　　　　　　　adj. 代谢的，新陈代谢的

metabolism [mə'tæbəlɪzəm]　　　　　　　n. 新陈代谢

microcirculation　　　　　　　　　　　　　n. 微循环

microprocessor ['maɪkrəʊˌprəʊsesə]　　　n. 微处理器

minimally invasive surgery　　　　　　　　微创手术

mobility [məʊ'bɪləti]　　　　　　　　　　n. 移动，机动性

molecular imaging　　　　　　　　　　　　分子成像

momentum [məʊ'mentəm]　　　　　　　　n. 动量

monocyte ['mɒnəʊsaɪt]　　　　　　　　　　n. 单核细胞

morphologic [ˌmɔ:fə'lɒdʒɪk]　　　　　　　adj. 形态的

morphometric　　　　　　　　　　　　　　adj. 形态测量的

motion sensor　　　　　　　　　　　　　　运动传感器

musculoskeletal & orthopedic biomechanics　肌肉骨骼与骨科生物力学

N

nasal splint　　　　　　　　　　　　　　　鼻夹

nebulizer ['nebjəlaɪzə]　　　　　　　　　　n. 雾化器

negative-pressure wound therapy　　　　　负压伤口治疗

nephrology and urology devices　　　　　　肾脏和泌尿系统器械

neurodegenerative dementia　　　　　　　神经退行性痴呆

neurology [njʊ'rɒlədʒi]　　　　　　　　　n. 神经学

neuromuscular [ˌnjʊərəʊ'mʌskjələ]　　　　adj. 神经肌肉的

neurostimulation	神经电刺激术
neurosurgery [ˌnjʊərəʊ'sɜ:dʒəri]	*n.* 神经外科（学）
neutrophil ['nju:trəfɪl]	*n.* 中性白细胞，嗜中性粒细胞
nitrogen ['naɪtrədʒən]	*n.* 氮气
nonactive medical device	无源医疗器械
nuclear medicine	核医学

O

obscuration bar	挡光棒，遮蔽条
occupational biomechanics	职业生物力学
ocular prosthetics	眼修复术
operative manipulation	手术操作
ophthalmic [ɒf'θælmɪk]	*adj.* 眼科的
ophthalmic device	眼科器械
optical microscopy	光学显微术
optical tracking	光学跟踪
optical-to-electronic coupling system	光电耦合系统
orthogonal [ɔ:'θɒɡənəl]	*adj.* 正交的
orthopaedic [ˌɔ:θə'pi:dɪk]	*adj.* 骨科的
orthopedic braces	矫形支架
orthopedic device	矫形器械
orthopedic implant	骨科植入物
orthopedic prosthetics	矫形修复学
oscilloscope [ə'sɪləskəʊp]	*n.* 示波器
osteoarthritis [ˌɒstiəʊɑ:'θraɪtɪs]	*n.* 骨关节炎
over-the-counter	*adj.* 无须处方可买到的，非处方的
oxygen bottle	氧气瓶

P

pacemaker ['peɪsˌmeikə]	*n.* 起搏器
pacemaker pulse generator	起搏器脉冲发生器
paramedic [ˌpærə'medɪk]	*n.* 急救医士
patella [pə'telə]	*n.* 髌骨
patella baja	低位髌骨
patellar tendon	髌腱
pathological processes	病理过程
pathology [pə'θɒlədʒi]	*n.* 病理学
perception [pə'sepʃən]	*n.* 知觉，感知

PET-CT scan	PET-CT 扫描
pharmaceuticals [ˌfɑ:mə'sju:tɪkəlz]	*n.* 药物
pharmacological [ˌfɑ:məkə'lɒdʒɪkəl]	*adj.* 药理学的
physical disability	残疾，肢体残疾
physiological process	生理过程
picture archiving and communication systems (PACS)	医学影像存档与通信系统
piezoelectric signal	压电信号
pigment ['pɪgmənt]	*n.* 色素，颜料
plantar-dorsiflexion	跖-背屈
platelet ['pleɪtlət]	*n.* 血小板
pleural wall	胸膜壁
ploidy analysis	（细胞）倍性分析
point-of-care testing (POCT)	即时诊断
position and orientation	位置和定向
positron emission tomography (PET)	正电子发射断层显像
post-operative [ˌpəʊst'ɒpərətɪv]	*adj.* 术后的
powered wheelchair	动力式轮椅
preoperative [pri'ɒpərətɪv]	*adj.* 术前的
projection radiography	放射照相术
proprioception [ˌprəʊprɪə'sepʃən]	*n.* 本体感受
prosthesis [prɒs'θi:sɪs]	*n.* 假体
prosthetic heart valve	人工心脏瓣膜
prosthetics [prɒs'θetɪks]	*n.* 假体（人造的身体部分），义肢
prototype ['prəʊtətaɪp]	*n.* 原型

Q

quadriceps tendon	股四头肌腱

R

radio frequency	射频
radiomics	*n.* 影像组学
radiotherapy [ˌreɪdiəʊ'θerəpi]	*n.* 放射治疗
radiotracer ['reɪdɪəʊtreɪsə]	*n.* 放射性示踪剂
receptor expression level	受体表达水平
reflectance photometer	反射光度计
refractive surgery	角膜屈光手术
registration [ˌredʒə'streɪʃən]	*n.* 配准
rehabilitation [ˌri:həbɪlɪ'teɪʃən]	*n.* 康复

rehabilitation engineering	康复工程
reproducibility [ˌriːprəˌdjuːsɪ'bɪlɪti]	n. 可重复性
research paper	研究论文
respiratory disposables	呼吸一次性用品
respiration pulse oximeter	呼吸脉搏氧饱和度仪
rheumatoid arthritis	类风湿关节炎
risk stratification	危险分层
robotic surgery suites	机器人手术套件
rule of thumb	经验法则，拇指规则，经验原则

S

sagittal ['sædʒɪtəl]	adj. 矢状的
saline solution	盐水溶液
sample stream	样本流
scapular ['skæpjələ]	adj. 肩胛的
scattered light	散射光
sensitivity [ˌsensə'tɪvəti]	n. 灵敏度
shaping ['ʃeɪpɪŋ]	n. 整形
sheath fluid	鞘液
short communication	短讯，研究简报
short-pass filter	短波通滤光片
side scatter (SSC)	侧向散射
signal conditioner	信号调理器，信号调节器
single-blind	单盲
skeleton ['skelətən]	n. 骨骼，骨架
socket ['sɒkɪt]	n. 接受腔，穴，槽，臼
sound hand	健侧手
spinal tap	腰椎穿刺
spirometer [spaɪ'rɒmitə]	n. 肺量计
sports biomechanics	运动生物力学
stem cell	干细胞
sterilization equipment and disinfectants	灭菌器械和消毒器械
stethoscope ['steθəskəʊp]	n. 听诊器
structural analysis	结构分析
stump [stʌmp]	n. 残肢
subcutaneous fat	皮下脂肪
submission procedure	投稿步骤

surgical container	外科手术容器
surgical dressings	外科敷料，外科用敷料，外科绷带
surgical instrument	手术器械
surgical navigation system	手术导航系统
surgical scissors	手术剪刀，外科剪刀
surgical sutures and staples	外科缝线和吻合器
suspend [sə'spend]	v. 悬浮
suspension [sə'spenʃən]	n. 悬浮液
syringe [sɪˈrɪndʒ]	n. 注射器

T

technical note	技术说明，技术注解
technical term	技术术语，专业术语
temporal resolution	时间分辨率
terminal device	终端设备
terminology [ˌtɜːmɪ'nɒlədʒi]	n.（某学科的）术语
theoretical basis	理论基础
therapeutic [ˌθerə'pjuːtɪk]	adj. 治疗的，医疗的，治病的
thermal ['θɜːməl]	adj. 热的，热量的
threshold ['θreʃhəʊld]	n. 阈值
tibia ['tɪbɪə]	n. 胫骨
tissue engineering	组织工程
tissue regeneration	组织再生
tomography [tə'mɒgrəfi]	n. 层析术，层析成像
tongue depressor	压舌板
total hip replacement	全髋关节置换
transducer [trænzˈdʒuːsə(r)]	n. 换能器，转换器
transfemoral ['trænsfemərəl]	adj. 经股的
transtibial	经胫骨的
trauma fixation	创伤固定（器）
treatment response evaluation	治疗反应评估
trigger ['trɪgə]	n. 触发器
tumor removal	肿瘤去（切）除
tumour hypoxia	肿瘤缺氧
two-color experiment	双色实验

U

ultrasound ['ʌltrəsaʊnd]	n. 超声波，超声，超声波扫描检查

urinary stone treatment	尿路结石治疗
urine analyzer	尿液分析仪

V

vastus lateralis obliquus (VLO)	股外侧斜肌
vastus medialis	股内侧肌
vastus medialis obliquus (VMO)	股内侧斜肌
vein thrombosis	静脉血栓
ventilator [ˈventɪleɪtə]	*n.* 呼吸机，呼吸器
venous return mechanism	静脉回流机制
virtual reality (VR)	虚拟现实
visual and tactile feedback	视觉及触觉反馈
volume, conductivity, and scatter	体积，电导，光散射

W

waterproof [ˈwɔːtəpruːf]	*adj.* 不透水的，防水的，耐水的
wearable sensor	可穿戴传感器
well-being assessment	健康评估
wheelchair [ˈwiːltʃeə]	*n.* 轮椅
working prototype	原型机
wound care	伤口护理
wound dressing	伤口敷料

X

X-ray	X 射线
X-ray machine	X 射线机

参考文献

[1] 刘蓉，齐莉萍. 生物医学工程专业英语[M]. 北京：电子工业出版社，2020.

[2] 陈秋兰. 医疗器械专业英语[M]. 第 2 版. 北京：人民卫生出版社，2018.

[3] 赵学旻. 医疗器械专业英语[M]. 上海：上海财经大学出版社，2015.

[4] Introduction to Flow Cytometry. https://www.thermofisher.cn/cn/zh/home.html.

[5] Bioengineering and Biomedical Engineering. https://engineeringonline.ucr.edu/.

[6] Bioengineering vs. Biomedical Engineering: Which is Right for You? https://blog.collegevine. com/bioengineering-vs-biomedical-engineering/.

[7] RAMAKRISHNA S, TEO W E, Tian Lingling, et al. Medical Devices: Regulations, Standards and Practices. Cambridge: Woodhead Publishing Ltd, 2015.

[8] MAHYUDIN F, HERMAWAN H. Biomaterials and Medical Devices. Switzerland: Springer International Publishing, 2016.

[9] 周剑涛. 检验技术专业英语[M]. 北京：人民卫生出版社，2015.

[10] Chinese Society of Biomedical Engineering. http://en.csbme.org/about/index.html.

[11] Arm Prosthesis. https://www.trsprosthetics.com/cybathlon-winner-bob-radocy/.

[12] Limb Prostheses. https://www.ottobock.lk/en/.

[13] Upper Limb Prosthesis. https://www.armdynamics.com/our-care/prosthetic-options.

[14] Lower Limb Devices. http://dukaortopedi.com/urun/ossur-rheo-elektronik-diz-eklemi/.

[15] Hematology Analysis. https://www.beckman.hk/.

[16] Medical Devices. https://www.ima.is/medical_devices/about_medical_devices/.

[17] Flow Cytometry. https://www.fishersci.com/us/en/brands/IIAM0WMR/invitrogen.html.

[18] FootFit Devices for Leg Ulcers. https://clinicaltrials.gov/ct2/show/NCT02632695.

[19] Introduction to Flow Cytometry. https://www.labome.com/method/Flow-Cytometry-A-Survey-and-the-Basics.html.

[20] Biomedical Signal Processing and Control. https://www.sciencedirect.com/journal/biomedical-signal-processing-and-control.

[21] KOWAL J, LANGLOTZ F, NOLTE L P. Basics of Computer-Assisted Orthopaedic Surgery. In: Navigation and MIS in Orthopedic Surgery. Springer: Berlin, Heidelberg, 2007.

[22] JARAMAZ B, DIGIOIA A M. (2004) CT-Based Navigation Systems. In: Navigation and Robotics in Total Joint and Spine Surgery. Springer, Berlin, Heidelberg.

[23] HEBECKER A. (2004) C-Arm-Based Navigation. In: Navigation and Robotics in Total

Joint and Spine Surgery. Springer, Berlin, Heidelberg.

[24] BENAZZO F, STROPPA S, CAZZAMALI S, et al. (2007) Principles of MIS in Total Knee Arthroplasty. In: Navigation and MIS in Orthopedic Surgery. Springer, Berlin, Heidelberg.

[25] WALKER P S, YILDIRIM G, SUSSMAN-FORT J. (2007) Implications of Minimally Invasive Surgery and CAOS to TKR Design. In: Navigation and MIS in Orthopedic Surgery. Springer, Berlin, Heidelberg.

[26] LAMBIN P, EMMANUEL R V, LEIJENAAR, et al. Radiomics: extracting more information from medical images using advance feature analysis. European Journal of Cancer. 48(4):441-446. doi: 10.1016/j.ejca.2011.11.036.

[27] Clinical Laboratory Science. https://clinicalsci.info/principles-of-automated-blood-cell-counters/.

[28] Human Factors and Medical Devices. https://www.fda.gov/.